How to Collect and Record a Health History

How to Collect and Record a Health History

Elizabeth Anne Mahoney, R.N., M.S.
Assistant Professor of Nursing

Laurie Verdisco, R.N., B.S., M.A.
Assistant Professor of Nursing

Lillie Shortridge, R.N., B.S., M.Ed.
Assistant Professor of Nursing

The Faculty of Medicine of
Columbia University
School of Nursing

J.B. Lippincott Company
Philadelphia
New York   San Jose   Toronto

Distributed in Great Britain by
Blackwell Scientific Publications
London Oxford Edinburgh

ISBN 0-397-54185-6
Library of Congress Catalog Card Number: 76-8712

Printed in the United States of America

2 4 6 8 9 7 5 3

Library of Congress Cataloging in Publication Data

Mahoney, Elizabeth Anne.
    How to collect and record a health history.

    Bibliography: p.
    Includes index.
    1. Medical history taking. 2. Medical records.
I. Verdisco, Laurie, joint author. II. Shortridge, Lillie, joint author. III. Title. [DNLM: 1. Medical history taking—Nursing texts. 2. Medical records, Problem oriented—Nursing texts. WY156 M214h]
RC65.M33   616.07'5   76-8712
ISBN 0-397-54185-6

TAbLE of CONTENTS

Acknowledgments

We would like to express our deep appreciation for the support and encouragement of our families, friends, and colleagues during the preparation of this manuscript. We wish to especially thank M. Rae Barone, who inspired us to publish materials on the health history, and Bernice Heller, Editor, J.B. Lippincott Company, for her advice and assistance in writing the book.

Sincere thanks are extended to the undergraduate students in the School of Nursing, Columbia University, who field tested the original programmed instruction on the Health History. Many of their suggestions have been incorporated in the book.

We are grateful to our friends and colleagues who reviewed portions of the manuscript and offered helpful comments.

We wish to thank Mary Bufi for her expert typing of the manuscript.

Elizabeth Anne Mahoney
Laurie Verdisco
Lillie Shortridge

March, 1976

pREfACE

The health care delivery system is the third largest industry in the U.S. In excess of $94 billion is spent yearly on all health services; over 7,000 hospitals provide patient care; suppliers of medical equipment and drugs number over 2,000; and insurance companies providing policies to 134 million persons number more than a thousand. There are over 4 million health care personnel, including 320,000 physicians and 800,000 nurses. Not only does the number of personnel continue to increase, so also do the categories. Nurse practitioners, physician assistants, dental auxiliaries, and various technicians function in a variety of ways toward client care.

Although each category of health care personnel has specific responsibilities, there are several areas of shared concerns. Among the most important of these areas is the assessment of the client: the collection and recording of pertinent data regarding the client that can be utilized by members of the health team in providing needed care. At present each member uses a form specific to his/her discipline, be it nursing, medicine, social service, physical therapy or nutrition, to collect data. These data may or may not be entered in detail in the client's chart or record. Similar data are collected by each of these persons, thus subjecting the client to multiple and often repetitive interviews. Frequently, it is necessary to search through the entire record and read several interviews before finding the needed information.

This book focuses on one aspect of assessment—the Health History. The Health History is the comprehensive account of the client's present and past wellness and illness. The format of the Health History presented in this book can be used by all those involved in direct client care: nurse, physician, medical or nursing assistant, social worker, chaplain, nutritionist, dentist, dental assistant, psychologist, physical therapist, occupational therapist. It is through such a comprehensive assessment that the health team is provided with the initial data which enable its members to plan and meet the client's needs.

The Health History format presented here is unique in that it can be used for any client, well or ill, and at any stage of the client's development. Most current literature on the Health History focuses on the person who is ill or on the use of different forms for the child or adult and various disciplines. The use of a single format by all personnel will establish baseline data; make the data more accessible and retrievable; decrease the need for multiple, repetitive interviews; facilitate cooperation among disciplines; establish common language for disciplines; allow for greater consistency in data collection and recording; decrease fragmentation of care; and allow the Health History to tell the story of the client. Thus, there are many advantages to a comprehensive format.

In Part I, the term "client's health history" is defined, and its value and components, and sources of data collection are described. Characteristics of oral and written communication, techniques for establishing an environment conducive to interviewing, specific interviewing procedures, and recording of data are discussed. Part II presents the individual components of the health history. Here, the emphasis is on the specific information to be elicited in each component and the kinds of questions to be asked in order to obtain the necessary data. Each chapter contains a summary in which key points are reviewed. Part III, Appendices, includes the Outline Guide for the Collection of the Health History, which may be used in data collection, and an example of two complete Health Histories. Study of this text should enable the learner to collect and record a Health History accurately and to feel confident about compiling meaningful data.

In the text, "he" is used throughout when referring to the client and "she" when referring to the history taker. Since a satisfactory alternative to these pronouns has not yet been invented, they are used for the sake of clarity. They have no other significance.

introduction to the health history

CHAPTER 1

OVERVIEW

All members of the health care delivery system are concerned with meeting the health care needs of clients. Although these needs are many and varied, the priorities can be summarized into three major goals of health care: the promotion of health, the prevention of illness, and the maintenance or restoration of health.

Health promotion refers to those activities of the individual, or related to the environment, which enable the person to utilize his energies and resources for constructive living. Practices such as eating a diet composed of the basic four food groups, the use of iodized salt and flouridated water, engaging in productive interpersonal relationships, all enhance the individual's life.

The prevention of illness involves identifying factors within the individual or the environment which can cause disease or injury (accidents) and taking appropriate measures. Such diverse factors as obesity, pathogenic organisms, chemical agents, and emotional tension may be involved. Examples of measures employed to prevent illness and its complications or injury due to these agents might include a reducing diet, adherence to a diabetic diet designed to prevent certain complications, immunization against a specific organism such as poliovirus, keeping medications and other chemicals out of reach of children, and alleviating or controlling stressful situations. You can see that teaching is an essential component in the prevention of illness.

The maintenance or restoration of health refers to cure or modification of disease or injury and return to an optimal although not necessarily a former level of living. Kinds of therapies or approaches which may be used to overcome illness or reduce its effects include: following a diabetic diet which is regulated according to the person's energy needs or insulin dose; taking an antibiotic for an infection; removing an inflamed appendix; receiving psychiatric help to cope with one's emotional problem; using a wheel chair or crutches for mobility.

The task of meeting health care needs may seem insurmountable when one considers the uniqueness of every person. How can anyone begin to know each client and his needs? The answer is that the needs of each client can be recognized through the individual and team effort of eliciting and recording factual information about him. This information, collectively called the data base, consists of three major parts: the health history, the physical examination, and the laboratory or diagnostic studies. When properly done, these combine to give health personnel an accurate understanding of the client. The health history is the first part of the data base—the foundation upon which the other two parts are built—and is the focus of this text.

Definitions

The terms *client, health,* and *history* are defined—first separately, and then collectively—to give us a common reference point.

A *client* is a consumer of services—any recipient of health care, regardless of the reason or setting. This broad definition includes the client who is ill and is receiving care—whether it be in the hospital, home, ambulatory care center, clinic, physician's office or place of employment—as well as the individual who is seeking promotive or preventive health care in a well-child clinic, early detection center, mobile unit, or the office of a physician, nurse, or social worker. Although the word "patient" is familiar and traditional, it has the negative connotation of illness; whereas "client" has much more scope and embraces all those people who seek and receive health care. It is important to appreciate this philosophy if you are to understand the Health History presented in this book.

The term *health* has many meanings, and is influenced by a variety of individual and cultural interpretations. Some describe health in a negative sense—the absence of sickness, pain, worries, need for a doctor. Others list the many positive factors which are indicative of "health" or "well-being"— eating well-balanced meals; attending school; productivity; participating in social and recreational activities; getting along well with others; living in adequate housing. The definition of health subscribed to in this text is the inclusive one which is stated in the Preamble to the World Health Organization Constitution in 1946: *"Health* is the state of complete physical, social and mental well-being and not merely the absence of disease or infirmity." This all-encompassing description of health clearly indicates that many facets of a client's life must be considered when planning or providing for his care. It is important to remember that an individual is not a static being but rather is constantly changing as a result of his interactions with other people and the environment. Health and illness are independent and contrasting situations; aspects of each in varying degrees can be present in one person, simultaneously. This is an important concept to consider in assessing a client—the focus cannot solely be on health or on illness, but must also allow for the potential presence of elements of each.

History, the final term, also has several definitions—even within a single dictionary. Two descriptions, very appropriate to this discussion, are found in the *Random House Dictionary of the English Language.* The first defines *history* as "a continuous, systematic narrative of past events as relating to a particular people, country, period, person, etc., and usually written in chronological order." The second refers to "acts, ideas or events that will or can shape the course of the future." History, for our needs, may be interpreted simply as the client's story of past and present events which may affect his current and future health status. Illustrations of the relevancy of historical data are as follows: 1) The age at which a child developed motor skills—is this consistent with the expected developmental patterns? 2) The present physical, home and work situations—are they potential sources of physical or emotional stress? 3) The past occurrence or current contact with measles for a woman in her first trimester of pregnancy—is there a danger of fetal malformation? 4) Other contacts with health facilities—does the client focus on health promotion or only on illness care? 5) A family history of sickle cell anemia—must the client be tested for this hereditary trait? These examples demonstrate that the client's history can tell many things.

Now that the words *client, health,* and *history* have been considered individually, they can be combined and defined as the term *client's health history.* The *client's health history* is the comprehensive account of his present and past wellness and illness—his personal story of health and sickness. The complete Health History must reflect knowledge of the client as a total person—a past and present physical, social, and emotional being.

Components

Since the purpose of the Health History is to provide pertinent information readily available to all members of the health team, it must be complete and in a logical sequence. One definition characterizes history as a "continuous, systematic narrative...." This systematic or logical approach provides for consistency and makes it easier to locate desired information. Regardless of who collects the Health History, specific data should be found at the same place in each history.

Thus, a format or guide is essential to insure a systematic approach and the inclusion of all pertinent data. The format for the Health History presented in this book has seven components. These components are:

1. Reason for Contact
2. Biographical Data
3. Current Health Status
4. Past Health History
5. Family History
6. Social History
7. Review of Systems

Each component will be explained briefly and then discussed in more detail in Part Two.

The *Reason for Contact* is a simple statment, in the client's own words, as to why he came to the health personnel and facility. This is the "why" of the contact. The reason may be promotion of health—"I came in for my routine physical examination"; prevention of illness—"Michael needs his polio vaccine"; maintenance or restoration of health—"I have a pain in my stomach."

The *Biographical Data* contain the client's "vital statistics": his full name and address; telephone number; age; date and place of birth; sex; ethnic group; religion; primary spoken language; marital, educational, and occupational status; health insurance; Social Security number; the first names of his parents and his mother's maiden name. This gives the health care personnel some general information about "who" the client is and what his background entails. It is a starting point in seeing the client as a total person; it gives direction to the interview, and can be significant in determining his health status.

The *Current Health Status* is a general impression of the client's state of health—a full description of his specific complaints, if applicable, and his daily habits and activity patterns. This provides an opportunity to identify not only "who" the client is, but also to get a general picture of his state of health.

The *Past Health History* relates data concerning the client's previous state of health or illness and his contact with health care personnel and facilities. This includes: developmental data; promotive and preventive practices; restorative interventions; allergies; and foreign travel.

The *Family History* involves data about the client's family composition, the present health status of each member, familial illnesses, and relationships existing among family members. This is important because the health of other family members affects the client just as his affects the family.

The *Social History* includes information concerning factors that influence the client's current life situation—relationships that occur outside the family, occupation/school, and environment. This component is concerned with the more personal factors regarding the client and his relations with others. It provides information concerning the client's social adjustment, and may indicate potential sources of illness in his physical and interpersonal environment.

The *Review of Systems* is the orderly assessment of the status of the major anatomical areas of the body. This is the final component of the Health History. It serves as an overall check that all relevant data have been obtained; the symptoms are grouped so that relationships among them can be seen more readily; and an opportunity is provided for the client to present more information than he initially communicated. This review is the informant's verbal response to questions about each system. The *Review of Systems* must not be confused with the physical examination. The areas of assessment are similar but the techniques used to obtain the data are different.

During collection of the Health History, opportunity should be provided for expression of the client's questions and concerns. Significant relative data should be included with the appropriate component. For example, a client states, "I twisted my right ankle six months ago but didn't feel medical help was necessary at the time." Although this is not his *Reason for Contact,* he states, "It still hurts a little when it rains. When do you think I can start playing tennis?" This information should be included in the *Current Health Status* where it was elicited, under Recreation and Exercise. Specific details of the injury would be included in the *Past Health History.* You may have noted some areas of potential overlap. Overlap is possible and to some extent built into the history. Redundancy is not intended; rather the purpose is to insure accuracy. Questions may go unanswered because they were unclear in the manner in which they were asked or the client may have forgotten data; yet when a similar item is asked later he suddenly understands or remembers. When you are interviewing a client regarding his *Past Health History,* for example, you may ask him if he has ever had surgery. He replies, "No." Later, under the *Review of Systems,* Integumentary System, you ask the client if he has had any skin lesions or growths. He responds, "I had a tumor on my arm; the doctor took it off in his office last May."

The placement of some data in two areas also may help to identify behavior patterns. For example, a client who usually does not seek attention when injuries occur may need counseling. Some repetition also serves as a check on the reliability of the informant. Is he consistent in his responses or is he confused or withholding data? All information does not need to be repeated in the record. For example, although the surgery described above was mentioned in the *Review of Systems,* it also should be recorded under the *Past Health History.* A notation is entered under the *Review of Systems,* Integumentary

System—"Data about tumor on arm are contained in the Past Health History."
The information has been included where it is necessary, not repeated in detail.

When the history is collected in the order presented, a logical sequence of information will result. Each person using the history will know the location of various data. Time is saved because personnel do not have to read through many pages to find the desired information, and they can readily determine whether all necessary facts have been included.

You may ask, why introduce another history format when there are so many forms already available—such as medical, nursing, and dietary—for collecting data about a client? There are almost as many forms as there are categories of health professionals or facilities! Each includes similar items, as well as specific ones for the particular discipline or group, with the result that the client is subjected to several interviews and repetitious questions while each worker is collecting information—yet none has a total picture of the client. Think for a minute of how you would feel if you had to repeat your name, age, and address to four different people during one visit to a health care facility. Think of Mr. Coyle, a 65-year-old man, recently retired, who is making his first contact with a Senior Citizen Center. There all new members are routinely interviewed by the health-assistant receptionist, social worker, nutritionist, and activities director on an individual basis, and each keeps her own records. Therefore, Mr. Coyle must repeat at least his name, age, and address to four people during one visit. One keeps statistics on new members and attendance; another seeks data on financial and housing needs; another is concerned with meal planning and food preferences; and the last with recreational interests. Mr. Coyle may respond with annoyance, boredom, frustration, or anger, and such reactions would be justified. This alone could be a reason for not seeking health care. Hence, both client and health personnel invest time and energy, gaining limited and fragmented results. There is no comprehensive account of the client's present and past wellness and illness.

Contrast that situation with this one: Mr. Coyle is investigating another Senior Citizen Center with similar facilities. The health assistant greets Mr. Coyle and begins to collect data, explaining their use in a Health History. The form is only partially completed when Bingo is to begin. Mr. Coyle has indicated a desire to participate in this and will later see the activities director. He leaves for Bingo, then sees the activities director, who now has the partial history. Mr. Coyle discusses his interests and gives information to complete the form. The completed Health History is reviewed and placed in a shared file. If Mr. Coyle needs nutritional, social service, or further recreational counseling, his "picture as a person" is readily available to all health personnel. He will not have to repeat his entire life story before his needs can be met!

A Health History eliminates redundancy and frustration, and effectively utilizes the client's contact with health personnel. All members of the team participate in the client's health care, yet a minimal number of history forms is required. Chapters to follow describe how the health history presented in this text can be used for any client, well or ill, at any stage of his development, by the entire health team.

Sources

By definition the Health History is the story of the client. Therefore, the client is usually the primary informant or source of information. However, at times, it may not be possible to obtain all or any of the necessary data from the client. The client may be an infant; a person who is forgetful, confused, or unconscious; or someone who is unable to speak or speaks another language. Thus, it is important to identify sources, other than the client, that can provide reliable data. These additional sources may include: relatives, friends, health team members who are familiar with the client, and the client's past records or charts. It is important to remember the potential sources of information about a client, so that they can be used when necessary. Even when the client is the primary informant, alternate sources such as charts or personnel can decrease the need for asking repetitious questions of the client and his relatives and friends, or records can help recall a forgotten event. A few situations will illustrate the use of available sources for data collection. Mr. Coyle was the primary and, initially, the sole source of information, as he came alone to both settings and was unknown to the health personnel and facilities. However, once the data were compiled in the second agency, the personnel and his record became additional resources for subsequent visits.

In another situation, Jimmy Robinson, age 3 years, comes to the Well-Child Clinic with his mother for a physical examination. As his family has just moved to the area, this is his first visit to the clinic. Here, Jimmy and Mrs. Robinson are the only available sources for data collection. Although Jimmy is the client, because of his age Mrs. Robinson is considered the major informant. Again, after this initial visit two other sources are available—the clinic personnel and his chart.

In contrast, Mrs. Delancey, a 70-year-old woman, accompanied by her husband, is returning for her monthly visit to the Diabetic Clinic of the hospital where her disease was initially diagnosed, and where she has been treated for the past 5 years. She has many sources of information readily available—herself, her husband, hospital personnel, records, and perhaps friends or acquaintances she has made in the clinic.

These examples show how a variety of resources—client, relative, friends, health personnel, and records—may be available and used to compile a total picture of the client. If additional sources of information are available and utilized, there is usually less chance of omitting pertinent data and a more accurate history is therefore obtained.

The foregoing situations also demonstrate that the Health History is usually collected on the client's first contact with the health care personnel and facility and is written on the client's record. Ideally, serial or ongoing data related to all the components should be collected on subsequent visits, regardless of the setting, and used to update the history. This necessitates the sharing of client information both within and between health personnel and facilities. Certainly this sharing should be easier to accomplish when the client returns to the same facility, but sharing among facilities should be encouraged as well.

There has been much discussion about the use of a centralized computer for storage of client data and easy recall. This potential centralization and accessibility of data underscore the importance of maintaining the client's individuality and protecting his privacy in any situation. He should not be made to feel that he is only a "number" and "facts" punched into a machine. The second area of concern is privacy—all data obtained from the client are confidential. This means that the Health History is collected and used by appropriate health team members for the welfare of the client. Many clients are hesitant to divulge personal factors for fear that the information may be misused. The client has the right to privacy—to know who will share the information and what safeguards are available to him to insure this privacy. Therefore, each health care worker has the responsibility of assuring the client that his permission is to be obtained before confidential data are disclosed and that only duly authorized persons will have access to the record.

Authorized personnel must use discretion when discussing the client's data. Here are some typical situations involving use of client data, analyzed in terms of maintaining confidentiality. Over a cup of coffee in the snack bar, a nurse and a social worker discuss John Hayes's financial status and his need for Social Service intervention. They are authorized personnel who have rightful access to the information and are using it for the welfare of the client. They have not, however, observed all necessary safeguards to maintain his privacy, and are violating his right to confidentiality by mentioning his financial (personal) status in a public setting and by using his full name. Unfortunately, this is a common occurrence. Unthinkingly, perhaps, personnel tend to discuss client's care in "nonsheltered" environments, such as coffee shops, elevators, and hallways. This is a disservice to the client involved as well as to all potential clients who would not want their information revealed so carelessly.

In comparison, a nursing team (RN's, LPN's, and assistants) discusses Mrs. Ruth Charles's present health status, in the conference room, for the purpose of planning her systematic care. The team members are authorized personnel who have legitimate access to her data and are using these to plan her care. As in the first situation, the client's name is used, but here the setting is a restricted environment—the conference room. It is appropriate to use Mrs. Charles's name so that all know to whom they are referring and, since the information is restricted to those in the conference room, unauthorized persons have no access to the data. Privacy is maintained because specific criteria and safeguards have been observed.

Frequently specific data are used in case studies for submission as course requirements or articles or for presentation at conferences. The full name of the client, family, and health personnel or facility may be used only with the permission of each individual subject involved. It is preferable and commonplace to identify any of these by the use of initials or pseudonyms or to keep them nameless. Such precautions protect the subject's identity. The audience or reader may be considered "authorized personnel in a learning situation." The client and/or others can benefit from this sharing of data, directly or indirectly in terms of immediately improved care or alternate approaches to care. Information is not misused, and privacy can be maintained.

The foregoing examples illustrate how a client's privacy can be preserved or violated. It is the responsibility of each person involved to respect the client's right to privacy and to adhere to all safeguards when confidential information is used. A client will divulge personal information more easily when personnel demonstrate that they are worthy of his trust.

Summary

The Health History is a comprehensive account of the client's *present and past health* which is used by all team members to plan and meet the client's needs. Data may be collected from any client *well* or *ill,* at any *stage* of development, by use of these seven components:

1. Reasons for Contact
2. Biographical Data
3. Current Health Status
4. Past Health History
5. Family History
6. Social History
7. Review of Systems

This format eliminates the need for numerous forms, and the data can be provided by several sources: client, relatives, friends, health team members who are familiar with the client, and client records.

The collection and recording of the Health History data afford exciting and challenging experiences to health personnel. Since the Health History is the foundation upon which all other health assessment is made, it must be as complete as possible. It is on the basis of Health History data that decisions are made as to the need for teaching, counseling, or referral. The Health History data also serves to direct personnel toward a thorough assessment during the physical examination and diagnostic studies. For example, a client states that he has been experiencing fatigue, weakness, and irritability. Upon assessment his diet is found to be low in iron. Since inadequate iron intake can cause anemia, a decision can be made that he needs dietetic education. The data also direct health personnel to examine the condition of the client's skin and mucous membranes, nails, tongue, and heart and to order specific blood tests to further define the anemia. Regardless of who does the teaching or performs the physical examination or laboratory tests, the person who collected the Health History has made an important contribution toward meeting the client's needs. She has provided the foundation upon which other data can be built. Hence each member of the team has the opportunity to become a "health detective," gathering all the significant "evidence" needed for a decision about the client's state of health and necessary care.

Since this may be the client's first contact with the health care delivery system or with a specific agency, every member of the health team has the opportunity not only to be a "health detective" but also to communicate interest in and concern for the client's well-being. She does this by introducing the client to the agency, setting the tone for subsequent client-personnel interactions, and communicating interest in and concern for him as an individual. Furthermore, she meets and interacts with many people, thereby increasing her ability to understand people, their needs, and their concerns.

CHAPTER 2

collecting the data

Effective communication is the basis for data collection. Communication may be defined as the exchange of or the imparting of thoughts, feelings, ideas, and information orally, in writing, or by signs, such as gestures or pauses, all of which find expression in the interview, the printed form, or the computer printout. Of these, the first means—the interview—involves personal, direct contact between the client and interviewer, whereas the others are vehicles of impersonal communication involving the client and a piece of paper or machine. Each method has its merits, advantages, and disadvantages.

Means of Communication

The interview is a formal, oral exchange of information and feelings, through which data are obtained. It is similar to conversation in that both involve the spoken word, and different from conversation in that the interview is formal while conversation is informal. An interview is sometimes called "conversation with a purpose."

Because it is based on personal, direct contact between the client and the interviewer, the interviewer has opportunity to guide the discussion toward appropriate topics while simultaneously establishing a relationship with the client by expressing interest and concern. At this time she can also observe the client's nonverbal responses—his gestures, posture, facial expressions, pauses, and topic changes. However, the very personal nature of the situation can hinder as well as facilitate communication. A climate conducive to sharing information is essential. The interviewer may either verbally or nonverbally, either consciously or unconsciously, demonstrate that she is neither interested in nor sensitive to what the client has to say. She may remind the client of someone from the past with whom he has had conflict; his present reactions may be based on those past experiences. Also, because of the face-to-face contact, the client may feel uncomfortable about divulging personal information for fear of reprisal or rejection. The interview can also be time-consuming for both the client and the interviewer.

A printed form can save time for both parties. It allows the client to proceed at his own pace, and it can be completed at home as easily as in the health care setting. Completing it at home affords time and resources for checking the accuracy of dates and other needed information. A printed form may lend objectivity or impersonality which the client may feel makes it easier for him to reveal personal matters—he fears no immediate reaction. However, the questions must be specific and clearly stated, in language appropriate to all levels, so that no confusion exists in the client's mind. He must be able to read and write the language or have resources available so that all data can be obtained. A client may react negatively to the impersonality of a form, feeling that it is robbing him of his individuality, or that he is reduced to being merely a name on a paper—not a person—with no opportunity for immediate feedback or support.

How might the client respond to a computer? He must be able to use the machine. How will he manage problems of a mechanical nature? He may actually have a fear of the apparatus. He may regard it as a threat to his privacy. On the other hand, the ease of access is an asset to the facility, and ultimately benefits the client by affording sharing of data. It may be possible to program the computer in such a manner as to decrease the impersonality of history taking. Some clients may really enjoy working with the computer.

Although all these methods have a place in Health History collection, the focus of this chapter is on the interview—the oral exchange of information between client and worker. The emphasis is on the interview because it is the one most often used: it promotes personal contact and both nonverbal and verbal communication. The interview is the bedrock for providing effective health care in all situations, whatever the setting. Then, too, it is not always feasible to employ printed forms or computers, because of a lack of time or equipment, or in emergency situations; and when these are utilized, subsequent personal contact still is necessary. Indeed, they supplement rather than replace the interview. Once information has been collected and reviewed, results are discussed with the client, further data can be obtained, and plans can be formulated.

Characteristics of Oral Communication

Since the interview is a means of oral communication, it might be helpful to describe what is meant by effective oral communication. Oral communication should be clear and understandable, frank and open, free flowing, relaxed, and flexible.

Clear, understandable comunication

Each person is aware of what the other is saying. There are no ambiguities or hidden meanings; a common language is spoken. The interviewer must identify the client's level of understanding and then proceed to phrase her comments and questions accordingly. However, this does not mean that the interviewer must completely adopt the client's words, slang, or "street" language; rather, she conveys appreciation of what he is saying or trying to say and phrases her thoughts accordingly. Her vocabulary is appropriate to the situation. The client who understands technical terms should feel as comfortable with the interviewer as one who has a limited vocabulary. Neither should feel that he is being talked down to or up to.

Frank, open communication

Friends are usually straightforward and sincere in their conversation. Although the interview is not an informal discussion, it must take place in an atmosphere of openness to insure that all necessary data will be expressed and that information will not be deliberately withheld. There are times when a client may hesitate to be candid, especially about deeply personal matters: his innermost feelings, anything that may cause embarrassment, or things he feels the interviewer may not wish to hear about. It is in these situations especially that a nonjudgmental attitude of sincere interest is vital. It can make the difference between encouraging and impeding verbalization. The interviewer establishes the basis for trust. She must communicate that she is there to promote the client's well-being, that she is concerned about him as a person, and that his privacy and feelings will be respected. The topic is discussed further on p. 19.

Effective oral communication ususally is free flowing and relaxed, making conversation easy, smooth, and free of uncomfortable pauses and tension. Ideally, the interview should be the same. However, circumstances sometimes inhibit such "ideal communication." Some subjects will by their nature be anxiety provoking—deep feelings, social patterns, family matters. It is the responsibility of the interviewer to minimize stress on the client, while still obtaining the necessary data. Again, through establishing trust and understanding, and by demonstrating sensitivity, this is possible, although it may take time to accomplish. Regardless of the *Reason for Contact,* seeking services for health care may evoke feelings of fear. The client may be very anxious or embarrassed by his need for health care; he craves help yet fears what may lie ahead and what may be required of him. His ability to communicate freely may be inhibited. The interviewer can help him to relax by her calm and unhurried manner or by saying something such as:

> Coming to the doctor's office can make one feel nervous.

She is communicating sensitivity by being nonjudgmental and by giving the client an opportunity to verbalize his concerns.

Oral communication is usually flexible, and it should be, within limits, during the interview. A flexible approach allows the client to proceed at his own pace and discuss his own perception of health priorities. Frequently the end result is more information than might be obtained from structured questioning. He senses that the interviewer is interested in him and in what he has to say. However, if he does digress widely, she must guide him back to the focus of the meeting.

At this point, you may question whether and how flexibility is compatible with the sequence of health history components. Certainly there can be flexibility as far as the data within each component is concerned; if the client moves on to information relevant to another component, the data can be stored for later reference and recording or pursued immediately. For example:

> Mr. Thomas is telling you about his stomach pain, its onset and duration. He also mentions that his wife "caught the flu a week ago" and later that "she still has it." Then he states, "I drink milk which eases the pain—but since my wife caught the flu, she gets sick every time she drinks milk."

Mr. Thomas seems very concerned about his wife's condition. He has mentioned it three times within a very brief period. His present needs might be better handled if he could verbalize further about his wife's health and his concern.

Your response:

> Mr. Thomas, you seem very upset. Tell me what is bothering you.

or

Mr. Thomas, you seem very concerned about your wife. (Pause)

In the first response, Mr. Thomas can choose that which concerns him: his stomach pain, his wife's condition, or perhaps something else. You have communicated interest and have given him the opportunity to talk freely about his concern. In the second response, you still have indicated sensitivity to what he is saying but you have chosen the focus—his concern for his wife—and therefore set a limit. If his wife's condition concerns him, he should talk about it. However, if he has another major concern, he may not feel free to discuss it at this time.

Both responses may elicit data relevant to the *Family History*, although the initial focus was his *Current Health Status*. After he has verbalized his concern, you can return to the subject of his current state of health and later record the information under the appropriate component.

However, a lack of sensitivity to other than his physical needs may be conveyed by ignoring his frequent references to his wife. A comment such as:

Mr. Thomas, tell me more about how you relieve your pain.

omits any mention of his wife. Likewise, you may recognize but postpone the client's verbalization of his concerns:

Mr. Thomas, tell me more about how you relieve your pain. We'll talk about your wife later.

Remarks such as these can influence the remainder of the interview. Mr. Thomas may relate to you only facts about his physical state. You may have communicated the notion that you have not listened to or are not interested in his description of his feelings. Later it may be difficult for you to convince him that you *are* concerned about him as a total person.

Formality

The interview has the added dimension of being a formal meeting. This does not mean that it has to be "stiff," "rigid," or "cold." It is a professional conversation rather than social chit-chat. The client has come to you or the facility for a specific purpose; he is a consumer of your services. You and the facility have something special to offer which is not readily available from his family or friends. Therefore, your respective roles have been set and should be adhered to, with respect for one another as individuals. Such may seem difficult, if not impossible to maintain at times, especially with a client who is openly hostile. How do you communicate respect yet preserve your objectivity? Recognize that while you are the recipient of the hostility, you are not its cause. Hostility may be a manifestation of anxiety. Thus before the interview can proceed, the client must be helped to deal with his hostility. One approach is to communicate your awareness of his anger and give him an opportunity to talk about it.

Mr. Chapman, you seem angry—tell me more about the way you feel.

You are acknowledging his feeling and providing him with an opportunity to verbalize and explore it; rather than confronting him with anger or a judgmental attitude. Once he can deal with his hostility, you can proceed with the collection of the history.

The interview is not the place to pass the time of day or discuss the weather. Both you and the client are meeting for a purpose—his health care—and *that* should be the topic of discussion. However, if a client appears very anxious or tense, a brief chat about the weather or the book he is carrying may help him to relax, and is appropriate. This may minimize his anxiety and make it easier for him to participate.

Climate

The interpersonal and physical environment must be such as to provide an atmosphere conducive to establishing rapport. It should foster a sense of ease so as to allay an anxiety he may have.

If the client has made an appointment for a complete physical examination and the Health History is to be collected at that time, he should be informed that each will take approximately 45 minutes to an hour, and this should be affirmed when he arrives for the appointment. The client who comes in without having made an appointment should be informed of the approximate length of the interview. In either case, the client is prepared—he knows that he will have sufficient time to discuss his health and any questions related to it.

Structuring the physical environment must take into account the client's physical comfort. If, for instance, he tells you that he is having pain, you must make him physically comfortable before proceeding with the interview. Is he having abdominal pain? He may find it easier to answer your questions if he is lying on his side with his knees and hips flexed, rather than sitting in a chair. If a couch or a bed is not available, sitting in a chair with his feet supported by a stool may provide some relief. Is he having back pain? He will be more comfortable and will find it easier to respond if he is sitting in a straight-back chair. Remember that the intensity of his pain may change. Initially, it may be minimal or tolerable but during the interview may intensify; you may have to stop the interview. Besides making the client more physically comfortable, this measure communicates your interest in and sensitivity to his needs.

A child may be more comfortable when toys, books, small chairs, or other familiar objects are available to him. He may be offered a pencil and a piece of paper, or some object that he can handle with safety. Thus, the child can remain close to the person who accompanied him, talk with the interviewer, and play. A more relaxed environment has been achieved.

The setting must be free from multiple interruptions so you can give your undivided attention to what the client is saying. Phone calls or undue noise may indicate to the client that your interests are elsewhere and that you are too busy to listen. The trust which may have been developing is negated by nonverbal communications from the physical environment which you have allowed. Interruptions create confusion, may necessitate repetition of questions, and may cause you or the client to lose the train of thought. Stimuli or activity can make for confusion; the client may forget important data.

Privacy is essential. Ideally, the room should be a closed one, away from noise. It should be well lighted, well ventilated, and equipped with comfortable chairs. Admittedly, it is not always feasible to have the "ideal" physical environment. At times the Health History may have to be collected on a busy hospital ward or in a crowded clinic, where private rooms are nonexistent or scarce. A curtain or partition, separating the bed or patient areas, may afford the only privacy. Since available resources must be utilized, the curtain is closed; a chair is drawn close; voices are as low-pitched as possible; within reason, privacy is maintained. Most clients will respond positively to sincere efforts of health personnel to provide the requisite environment, though the results may be less than optimal.

Establishing rapport is the basis for trust and for a productive interview that is mutually satisfactory. Your approach to the client and your questions must be carefully thought out, and should reflect consideration of his background. Remember that you are encouraging the client to discuss extremely personal matters, and he may feel threatened. It is the health personnel who set the climate and tone of the interview. The client is the "guest" or the "outsider" unless the meeting is held in his home. You are in your own domain and have control of the situation. Your initial greeting should be friendly, conveying a feeling of warmth, genuine concern, and interest. These feelings should be reinforced throughout the interview. So often, it is not what is said, but how it is said, that "turns the client on" or "off." It is difficult to generate trust in an atmosphere charged with abrupt, condescending, unconcerned, impersonal, or judgmental attitudes. Be relaxed, unhurried, encouraging, and acceptive of what the client has to say—the client will feel free to express his feelings openly without fear or censure.

The focus of the interview must be on the client—this is his story. It is disconcerting to be talked at during the meeting, or to watch the interviewer concentrate on note-taking rather than on what one is saying. You can write the history when the interview is completed.

The interpersonal climate—the verbal and nonverbal communication—is the essence of the interview. The verbal communication gives content as well as feeling tones, while nonverbal communication basically conveys feelings and attitudes. Is the client or interviewer happy, angry, interested, bored, fearful, insensitive, denying, avoiding? All of these and more may be identified by the perceptive observer whether he/she be client or health personnel. A gesture, a smile, a frown, fidgeting, an erect posture, a slump; they all tell you something. A pause, a silence, a change of topic can say, "I am unsure, let me think; I am uncomfortable with what we are saying, let's not talk about it." The task is to use all of the cues—verbal and nonverbal—so that communication is facilitated.

Stages of the Interview

The interview may be divided into three major stages: the beginning, the data collection, and the termination. Begin by introducing yourself. Use proper names; identify your role and the purpose of the interview.

> Good morning, Mr. Jones, I am Miss Thomas, a nurse. I shall be asking you some questions about your health.

If the client is a child, use his first name. It is advantageous to discover if the child has a nickname which he prefers; using it will make him more comfortable. Once the client is seated in a conducive environment, the Reason for Contact may be elicited through an open-ended statement such as:

> Mr. Jones, tell me why you have come.

The data collection proceeds with the interviewer using a variety of interviewing techniques, both verbal and nonverbal.

The termination includes a conclusion, possibly a summary and plan. A sample termination is:

> *Interviewer:* Mr. Jones, I am through with my questions. Do you have any questions or is there anything else you would like to talk about?
> *Mr. Jones:* No—I can't think of anything else.
> *Interviewer:* Then I shall begin your physical examination. You can change into a gown in the dressing room.

This termination has prepared the client for the end of the interview, as opposed to an abrupt:

Interviewer: Now I shall do your physical examination.

In the first situation, the end comes as no surprise. The client has had opportunities to ask questions or to discuss what is important to him and, perhaps, what he has hesitated to mention earlier. The second interview ends without any forewarning. The client has had no opportunity to ask questions and does not even know if all of the necessary information has been collected.

The summation is a brief statement of what has been accomplished and usually reemphasizes the purpose of the meeting. The plan gives direction for the future—teaching, consultation with other health team members, need for physical examination, diagnostic tests, and other measures. Sometimes, it may be less specific than described above, until all the data have been collected and the client's needs have been identified.

Interviewing Techniques

A variety of interviewing techniques exist. Their purposes are to encourage verbalization, to facilitate data gathering, and to establish productive interpersonal relationships. So many techniques are available that it will be useful to discuss them under the broad headings of directive and nondirective interviewing. Examples will be used to demonstrate their relevance to the Health History.

Directive techniques are those which give specific focus or direction to the topic under discussion. "Tell me more about your wife's flu." "Which leg bothers you?" "How old are you?" "Did Tommy walk alone before his first birthday?" "You wince when you turn your head to the left, does it hurt you?" "Have you had anything like this before?" *Closed questions* or *statements, sequencing events, validating observations,* and *encouraging comparisons* are the commonly used forms of directive techniques. While they all may elicit pertinent data, they are usually limiting as to the extent of information the client will give because he may not feel free to elaborate. Directive techniques have their greatest value when specific factual data must be elicited; in clarifying what the client is saying; if time is limited; or when a client has difficulty in focusing or relating data and is not responding to nondirective techniques.

Nondirective techniques are those which allow the client to select or elaborate on a subject. *Silence* can communicate understanding and encouragement, when the interviewer leans toward the client in a nonthreatening manner and without distracting gestures. *Acceptance* is conveyed through the use of "yes," and "uh hum," both of which tell the client "I am listening, please continue." *Open-ended statements* and *questions*—"Go on," "Tell me what concerns you," or "What brought you here?"—provide the client with the opportunity to pursue the area of most concern to him. Reflection and restatement are two other frequently used nondirective techniques. *Reflection* brings back to the client the thoughts, feelings, or actions he is expressing. For example:

> *Mrs. Hendrickson:* I'm pregnant. I don't know how to tell my husband.
> *Interviewer:* You feel afraid to tell your husband you are pregnant.

The client's words and feelings have been rephrased. You are telling Mrs. Hendrickson what you heard without being judgmental, and the topic now can be pursued in any direction Mrs. Hendrickson wishes. *Restatement* is the repetition of the main idea being stated:

> *Paul:* I am not doing very well in school.
> *Interviewer:* You are having difficulty in school.

You are communicating interest and encouraging Paul to speak; and he can now elaborate on his "difficulty in school." The foregoing examples illustrate the common forms of nondirective interviewing.

Two interview approaches to the same client will illustrate how directive and nondirective techniques elicit similar and contrasting data for a *Reason for Contact.*

Interview 1

> *Interviewer:* What seems to be the problem?
> *Client:* My leg has been bothering me.
> *Interviewer:* What is it about your leg that bothers you?
> *Client:* A rash has developed.
> *Interviewer:* Where is the rash?
> *Client:* Oh, it's on the front of my leg—just below my knee.
> *Interviewer:* On which leg?
> *Client:* My right one.
> *Interviewer:* How long have you had this rash?
> *Client:* Oh, about two weeks, it doesn't seem to want to go away.

This interview started with a nondirective question, and then proceeded with a series of specific questions. The factual data for the client's *Reason for Contact* have been elicited effectively, in that data gathering has been facilitated and some verbalization has been encouraged. The establishment of a productive interpersonal relationship, however, cannot be evaluated at this time.

Interview 2

> *Interviewer:* What seems to be the problem?
> *Client:* My leg has been bothering me.
> *Interviewer:* Tell me more about it.
> *Client:* Well, I've developed this rash on my leg.

Interviewer: (Silence)—nods encouragingly to client.
Client: It started two weeks ago—here (points to right leg, one inch below the knee). At first it was small, like a dime; now it goes all the way down to my ankle. My wife told me to wash it twice a day with Epsom salts. I have been doing that, but it just won't go away—my wife's afraid she'll catch it.

The second interview has used verbal and nonverbal nondirective interviewing techniques. It has yielded the factual data for the *Reason for Contact,* plus the treatment which the client has instituted. It also reveals information about the client's wife, their relationships and possible concerns. He followed his wife's suggestion for treating the rash, and it may be concern (his or hers) for its spreading to her that motivated him to seek help. You can validate this by questioning the client. Certainly, this interview has elicited factual data, encouraged verbalization, and set a climate for productive interpersonal relations. The interviewer has said little orally, yet has obtained substantial data. The client has revealed those aspects of his *Reason for Contact* which are pertinent, in his own way and at his own pace.

Although these examples have emphasized a more supportive role of the interviewer using the nondirective approach, this can and should be an integral part of either approach. Likewise, both directive and nondirective techniques should be used in collecting the Health History; in fact some components lend themselves to a particular technique. You may find that you use more directive techniques when collecting the *Biographical Data* or *Review of Systems.* You may introduce each area with an open-ended statement or question, but follow with more focused questions. For example, you may ask a client to "tell me about yourself" to obtain *Biographical Data.* His response may include his name, age, birthdate and place, and marital and occupational status. However, you will still have to ask direct questions to obtain his address, phone number, hospitalization coverage, and Social Security number. Similarly, specific data for each system may not be volunteered initially under the *Review of Systems,* so some direction is necessary. The main cautions with directive techniques are that they not be overused, thus turning the interview into a question-answer session; that they are not so directive that the client is using your words and not his own; and that you are not receiving only "yes" or "no" responses.

Summary

Communication involves the exchange of thoughts, feelings, ideas and information, orally, in writing, or by signs. Data collection for the Health History can utilize all of these methods but the most extensively used is the interview, or formal oral communication. Effective oral communication is understandable, frank, free-flowing, and flexible. In addition, the interview is formal and professional in manner, and incorporates nonverbal communication. The interpersonal and physical environment provides the framework for the interview, and valuable health information is collected.

The interview should progress smoothly through three major stages: the beginning or introduction, the data collection, and the termination. Since the interview can be fatiguing for both client and interviewer, the Health History should be completed within 45 minutes to an hour. A blend of directive and nondirective techniques enables the interviewer to encourage the client to verbalize, facilitates data collection, and establishes productive interpersonal relationships.

chapter 3

RECORdiNÇ THE dATA

Since the Health History is to be used by all members of the health team, the data must be readily accessible and meaningful to these personnel. Although the information could be conveyed orally—to each member individually or on a tape recording—it is more efficient in terms of time, energy, and recall to put it in writing. Individual oral communication may be more personal by affording the opportunity to discuss the situation in depth; however, the data collector would have to repeat all of the necessary information piece by piece with each health team member. This would be time consuming, and repetitious. Then, too, her presence would be necessary whenever the data were needed, and to avoid omissions she would have to be capable of recalling all data for each client. This is an unrealistic expectation. Individual oral communication is not a feasible method for maintaining a permanent Health History, although it certainly has its role in planning for the specific health needs of a client.

The use of a tape recorder is a more practical means of oral communication. It can be made available to all members of the health team, it eliminates the need for repetition by the data collector, decreases the danger of forgetting communication, and serves as a permanent record. However, it also has some disadvantages. Special equipment—the recorder and tapes—is necessary and can be expensive. Data must be organized before being recorded. Specific information may also be difficult to locate. If a nurse wants to evaluate the client's dietary patterns, she must play the tape through the *Current Health Status* until that segment is reached. If additional data are needed, they also must be discovered on the tape. Using a recorder, the nurse would have to listen through the tape until she reached the *Past Health History;* she could then find out if he had any prior dietary problems. To complete her data collection she would then have to play the tape until she reached the Gastrointestinal System of the *Review of Systems*—certainly a time-consuming endeavor.

The written record is the most common and efficient method of transmitting permanent data. It is available to all health team members; eliminates the need for repetition by the data collector; decreases the danger of forgetting information; does not require costly equipment; and provides easy access to specific facts.

Although initially it will be more time consuming to relate the data for the Health History in *any format* while you familiarize yourself with the process and develop precision in dealing with it, writing becomes easier and takes less time as you gain experience. It is like learning to type. You may type slowly and with mistakes at first, but with practice you become skillful and improve your accuracy and speed. Similarly, with practice and experience, you will become more adept in recording a Health History.

In this chapter emphasis will be placed on the written record of the Health History since it is the most efficient method. The criteria are the same for a tape recording. The record must be dated and signed (with name and title) by the person conducting the interview. These provide essential reference points for the contents of this contact and subsequent ones.

Criteria for effective communication in the Health History are the same as for any written communication: it must be clear, understandable, legible, complete, orderly, consecutive, logical, concise, succinct, and factual. For ease of recall the terms have been combined into five major categories, each beginning with the letter "c": client's words, clarity, completeness, conciseness, and consecutiveness. Each term will be defined and examples will be given, to afford a common reference point.

Client's Words

The client's words should be used whenever possible; they are the most informative in that they convey his understanding of the situation; its meaning to him; his ability to recall events and to organize his thoughts and then communicate his knowledge and thoughts to others. The Health History is his story and should be as personal as possible. Open-ended statements or questions provide more opportunity for self-expression. The history taker should ask clarifying questions but should avoid using professional jargon, or making assumptions. The client's words should be recognized in the record; they can be paraphrased and be preceded by the terms "client says, states, denies, etc.," or placed within quotation marks if they are a direct citation. For example, a client is asked why he came to the clinic.

> *Interviewer:* Why have you come to the clinic?
> *Client:* My stomach hurts.
> *Interviewer:* Where does your stomach hurt?
> *Client:* Oh, here (points to umbilical area.) It feels like I ate a ton of bricks.

The dialogue clearly identifies the client as the informant. The recording of the data also must denote the specific client comments whenever possible. As with any written quotations, the client's or informant's direct comments are identified by use of quotation marks when they occur as phrases or short sentences or by indention of the statements on separate lines on the page(s). When the client's or informant's words occupy three or more consecutive lines, the statements must be indented.

The recording of the verbal and nonverbal client communication in the preceding interview would be similar to either of these:

> 1. Paraphrased: The client states that his "stomach" hurts," but points to the umbilical area. He says that it feels as if he ate a "ton of bricks."
> 2. Direct Quotation: "My stomach hurts" (but points to umbilical area). "It feels like I ate a ton of bricks."

These entries reflect the client's words. They readily identify his *Reason for Contact* and his perception of the discomfort. They also indicate a discrepancy between the client's verbalization of the location of pain and the exact site of discomfort. The term *stomach* frequently is used when abdomen is meant; therefore, the exact site must be located.

However, if the entry in this situation was recorded as:

> Client complains of heavy abdominal pain in the umbilical region, suggestive of bowel obstruction.

the writer has made one of many potential diagnoses but has based her judgment on assumption rather than fact. The purpose is to collect data, not to diagnose. Much has been lost in this translation—the client's perception and expression;

an objective approach to data collection; and accurate information from which other health team members can draw their conclusions.

Paraphrases or direct quotations also apply when the source of information is an agent other than the client. The informant must be identified and his words used whenever possible. Thus, when Mrs. Kosti is admitted to the hospital in an unconscious state and her husband is providing the information, this must be noted in the chart.

> 1. Paraphrased: Husband states that she has been vomiting coffee-like material for two days and has had nothing to eat for the past twenty-four hours.

or ...

> 2. Informant's words: "My wife has been vomiting coffee-like material for two days; she hasn't eaten anything for twenty-four hours."

Each entry indicates the informant is the husband, as his comments are paraphrased or directly quoted. If parents, relatives, friends, health personnel, or charts are the source of information, they too should be clearly identified. Then, should any question arise, the informant is identified easily and can be contacted for clarification.

Keep in mind that quoting the client's or informant's words sometimes gives rise to exceptions to principles of effective communication. It is permissible, in fact it is necessary, to use phrases, contractions, or diagnostic terms, if these are direct quotation of the client or informant. For example:

> 1. Client says: "I have not had a bowel movement in five days and my stomach hurts."
> 2. Client states: "Constipation; get it every month or so; enema is the only thing that helps; this time it didn't work though."
> 3. Mother states: "Timothy has pain and swelling in his pharynx. Could it be a peritonsillar abscess?"

Although contractions, phrases, and diagnostic terms have been used and the grammar is not precise, these are appropriate entries on the charts, because they are the client's or informant's perceptions and wordings and are identified as such. Thus, what may be inappropriate comments from the interviewer can be acceptable when from the client or informant.

Clarity

Clarity is a hallmark of effective communication. This criterion relates to the intelligibility, or preciseness and legibility of the record. Two major questions to ask yourself are: Is the thought easily understood? Can the handwriting be easily read?

Words should be specific; indefinite terms such as "good," "large," or "moderate" are subject to individual definition and should be avoided or further explained. For example, "Mr. Moriarity is in 'good' health" is a common yet vague statement. What is "good" health? What standards are being used? Who has labeled his health as "good"—the client or the interviewer? Do all persons agree on the meaning of "good"? From the discussion in Chaper 1, it is easy to see that health has a variety of connotations. Which is applicable here? Is "good" health freedom from overt disease? Productivity? Or is it physical, social, and mental well-being? Many questions have to be raised because the statement is unclear. A more precise entry would be:

> Mr. Moriarity states he is in "good" health. He has not missed a day's work due to illness in five years.

It is now known that the client has considered himself to be in good health. Everyone reading the record knows that Mr. Moriarity's criterion for being in a state of good health is being able to go to work. The remainder of the Health History will provide data to support or negate the accuracy of this perception in relation to the broader definition of health, but at least an initial frame of reference has been established.

Terms of quantity, such as "large," "moderate," or "small" can also be confusing. To a child, a man of 5 feet 9 inches is "large" or "big"; by American statistics he is of "average" height; yet he is "small" for a professional basketball player. Each description may be accurate to the individual's perception—but how can they be reconciled into a common definition? In this situation the common denominator is the height of 5 feet 9 inches. This figure is constant regardless of who is looking at the man. Thus, specific measurements should be used in recording whenever possible. A client states he he has a "small" red area on his leg. He is asked to describe it in more detail: Which leg? Where on the leg? Can he approximate the size in inches or in relation to an object? He states that the area is about the size of a nickel on his left inner ankle. Thus, the entry on the chart would read:

> Client describes "a small red area about the size of a nickel on my left inner ankle."

This statement is much clearer than:

> Client states he has "a small red area on my leg."

Everyone reading the first statement knows the client's perception of the location and size of the red area; there is no room for doubt.

Clarity of content also concerns the use of terminology which is meaningful to all health team members. Just as the client should understand the questions that he is being asked, so the health team should understand what they are reading. Therefore, uncommon terminology, abbreviations, and symbols should be avoided, and words should be explained. Each health care discipline has formulated a jargon—the unique terminology employed by its members which is immediately recognized and understood by them.

Abbreviations and symbols can be vexing and can make record reading a guessing game rather than a source of information. Since the record is a source of meaningful information, and because there is such diversity of abbreviations and symbols, some peculiar to a particular agency, *all* abbreviations and symbols should be avoided:

1. Mr. Jacobson, 45 y.o. referred by LMD to I.H.C. for CBC and ESR.
2. Mr. Jacobson is a 45 year old man who is referred to the Ideal Health Clinic by his local medical doctor for a Complete Blood Count and an Erythrocyte Sedimentation Rate.

Can you interpret the first entry? If you are unfamiliar with the abbreviations and symbols used, this could be an exercise in frustration. Would each member of the health team recognize these? Would the social worker or the chaplain? Has the writer communicated all pertinent information to the appropriate people? These are the questions which must be constantly kept in mind, if the record is to be effective. In both of the examples given the same information was communicated, but the second stated the data more clearly.

Appropriate grammar and spelling also fall in the category of clarity of content. There should be no question as to the wording of the record, as there should be no confusion about unfamiliar terminology, abbreviations, and symbols. "Look it up" in a dictionary if you are unsure of the spelling. Examine the following entry:

Mr. Hopkins sees his opthamologist when necessary and is dependent on glasses for close work.

What assumptions would you make? Does "sees" mean he visits his specialist for an examination or that he "sees" him professionally? Shall we interpret "when necessary" as his annual examination appointment or could it mean he has difficulty focusing on close work? Does "dependent on glasses" mean that he wears glasses? Finally, "opthalmologist" is misspelled. An acceptable revision of the information might read:

Mr. Hopkins is examined annually by his ophthalmologist, and wears glasses when doing close work.

The information is clearly stated; grammar and spelling are correct.

The second component of clarity is legibility; can the handwriting be read? Since most records are not typed, this is especially important. Printing is an alternative if your handwriting is poor. If the writing cannot be deciphered, no one will ever know if all of the foregoing components have been included or if the remaining criteria have been met.

The headings for the components and their subdivisions should be underlined for emphasis and easy location.

Completeness

The next criterion for effective communication is *completeness.* This refers to totality of content and sentence structure. The Health History is described as the "comprehensive account of the client ... reflecting knowledge of the client as a total person." Seven components have been identified to insure the inclusion of all pertinent data. All components and their specifics, which will be discussed in greater depth in Part Two, must be incorporated. The data must reflect positive and negative responses to questions and descriptions of the type, frequency, and extent of activities.

An initial check for completeness begins with verifying that the seven components of the Health History are included: *Reason for Contact, Biographical Data, Current Health Status, Past Health History, Family History, Social History,* and *Review of Systems.* If the answer is "yes," then you can proceed to look critically at each component. If the response is "no," you have identified the need to collect missing data. When the client or other sources of information are accessible you can gather the information at that time. If no source is available, then a note should be made on the record in a prominent place, such as the front of the chart, so that the person who has the next contact with the client or other source of data may collect the necessary information. An appropriate comment for the chart of a client who is being seen in the clinic:

Date

Social and Family histories are missing. Please collect them on next clinic visit.

Becky Lang, R. N.

A notation of the chart of Mr. Cope, who has given only a partial history before he goes to x-ray, is:

Date

A partial history was obtained from Mr. Cope before he went to x-ray. Please collect his Past Health History and Review of Systems.

Naomi Roseman, R. N.

Once you have ascertained that all of the components are present, you can begin to evaluate their thoroughness. Reference to Outline Guide, Appendix A, may be helpful during your initial history taking. Questions that may be asked in evaluating completeness are: Have all necessary data been collected for each area? Is there any doubt whether certain questions have been asked? Each specific area should carry comments, including both positive and negative responses. For example, the Family History contains a section relating to the occurrence of certain diseases in family members. The presence or absence of each disease must be noted:

> Client denies family history of diabetes mellitus, hypertension, blood disorders, gout, arthritis, obesity, allergies, epilepsy, heart disease, mental illness, renal disease, cancer, alcoholism, migraine, and the presence of jaundice or anemia.

When the information is noted in this manner, each person reading the history can be certain that each disease has been reviewed with the client; there is no need to doubt that one has been omitted. In contrast, the terse notation on another *Family History:*

> Familial diseases denied.

leaves much room for speculation. Is the client aware of what are considered familial diseases? Has the interviewer asked the specific questions? How accurate and complete is this section?

The reader should not have to make assumptions about what data have or have not been reviewed. The section of the *Family History* above is a common area for lack of completeness. Others are: (1) specificity of the client's daily habits in the *Current Health Status,* (2) acute infectious diseases, immunizations, and contacts with health care practitioners and agencies in the *Past Health History,* and (3) the entire *Review of Systems.* A few further examples will illustrate these common pitfalls.

Duncan and Greg are two preschoolers who have had their annual physical examinations. Duncan's record of immunizations indicates that he had the "usual childhood immunizations." Greg's chart states:

> He had diphtheria, tetanus, pertussis vaccine in 1970 (age 3–6 months), smallpox vaccine in 1970 (age 6 months), oral polio vaccine in 1970 (age 9 months), measles vaccine in 1971 (age 1 year). He has had no tuberculin skin test or immunization against mumps.

You can see at a glance that Greg's entry is much more complete.

Another aspect of completeness relates to the type, frequency, and extent of activities, and everyday situations. These provide information about life style, patterns of health care, and areas such as developmental progress. For example:

> He walks two miles a day and plays tennis, indoors and outdoors, approximately two times a week.

This, as opposed to the terse statement "I exercise regularly," gives more specific information.

It is also important to note the frequency of contacts with health care practitioners and facilities. Under the *Past Health History* or *Review of Systems*—Mouth and Throat—you enter not only the last dental visit, but also the frequency of visits:

> He has had dental checkups every 6 months; the last examination was 3 months ago. He had no cavities last year.

or

> His last dental exam was 5 years ago. He feels no pain, so does not see the need to visit the dentist.

Both entries provide valuable data for health personnel. The first note indicates that the client recognizes the value of preventive health care and seeks services even when no problems are present. The second client has communicated a lack of orientation to preventive care and most likely seeks only curative care; he presents a need for health teaching which will be substantiated, most likely, in other parts of the history.

Once thoroughness of content has been ascertained, the writer must focus on completeness of sentence structure, i.e., phrases and contractions are avoided. Are the sentences grammatically correct? Avoidance of abbreviations has been discussed under *Clarity;* here the reference is to the elimination of contractions. The history should read as smoothly as a story.

Many personnel argue that it is unnecessary and time consuming to write sentences; that phrases are adequate, and that in practice, phrases are used in writing histories. Most authorities agree that the history should be written in complete sentences for ease in reading and for clarity. There is then no doubt as to who or what is the subject, for the record is more personal. Even those who do not practice this rule affirm its value and encourage others to implement it. It is just as easy to write under the *Review of Systems:*

> Mr. Lawrence has had no headaches or head injuries.

as it is to write:

> No headaches; no head injuries.

Conciseness

Conciseness calls for a record that is a brief story—short and to the point. Lengthy narratives can be boring; the reader loses interest; and they can unwittingly mask or omit pertinent data. However, completeness must not be sacrificed for brevity. Several excerpts from *Biographical Data* will illustrate:

> 1. Tony Palermo is a five year old boy. He is Caucasian. Born in New York City, he now resides there with his parents. His parents are second generation Italian-Americans.
> 2. Tony Palermo, a five year old boy, is Caucasian and a third generation Italian-American. He was born, and continues to reside, in New York City with his parents, Mary (nee Brown) and John.
> 3. Tony Palermo—a 5 year old Caucasian boy. 3rd generation Italian-American. Born and lives in New York City with parents, Mary (nee Brown) and John.

The first example contains most of the pertinent data, with the exception of parents' first names; however, it is not recorded briefly. The first two sentences are short and choppy, while the last sentence is a description of the parents rather than of Tony.

The second recording is concise—brief and complete. Relevant data concerning age and racial and ethnic background have been combined; his place of birth and residence and parents' first names are stated succinctly.

The last excerpt is brief, but completeness has been sacrificed for conciseness. Although the content is complete, telescopic language has been used in place of complete sentence structure.

Initially it may be difficult to write concisely, but practice leads to skill, a feeling of accomplishment, and satisfaction through effective communication.

Consecutiveness

The final "c"—*Consecutiveness*—refers to the logical presentation of the data. Each component and its subsequent parts follow the others in order and without omission. This provides for a consistent, organized approach that facilitates smooth reading throughout the history; thus, particular components can easily be located. Specific data should be found in the same place in each history as was stated in Chapter One. Thus, the seven components follow in orderly sequence, beginning with *Reason for Contact* and ending with the *Review of Systems.* Each *Review of Systems* begins with general information concerning the client's weight, height, and well-being, then progresses through each system and ends with Allergic and Immunologic Conditions.

The client may relate information that should be recorded later in the Health History.

Mrs. Farrell has come to a new physician for a flu injection. She states that she had pneumonia three years ago and is now "very susceptible to colds." She presents with no cough, or dyspnea, but wants the "shot as a preventive measure because the flu season is beginning."

The data are pertinent to three different components of the history, although they were all stated at one time:

Mrs. Farrell wants "a flu shot as the flu season is beginning"—*Reason for Contact.* She "had pneumonia 3 years ago" (1972) and is now "very susceptible to colds."—*Past Health History.* She presents with "no cough or dyspnea"—*Review of Systems: Respiratory.*

When the data are recorded, they are organized appropriately and written in sequence. Thus, entries would appear under:

Reason for Contact: Mrs. Farrell wants "a flu shot as the flu season is beginning."
Past Health History: She "had pneumonia 3 years ago" (1972) and is now "very susceptible to colds."
Review of Systems: Respiratory: She presents with "no cough or dyspnea now."

Relevant information has been obtained and recorded in a logical manner, and at the same time the client has had freedom of expression and was not interrupted as she communicated data about her status.

Other circumstances such as an emergency situation or a fatigued client may preclude collecting all the data at one time or in order. The information, however, should be organized and recorded in sequence, with notations concerning the omissions, so that ultimately the history will be consecutive and complete.

Summary

The written record is the most common and efficient means of permanent data transmission. The writing of the Health History was the focus of this chapter. The criteria also apply to tape recording. The five "c's," or characteristics of effective data transmission and recording, were identified: the client's or informant's words, clarity, completeness, conciseness, and consecutiveness.

The client's or informant's words should be used whenever possible. They are identified by statements such as, "client states," or "mother says" when data are paraphrased. Quotation marks indicate direct citations; indentions signify quotes of three or more lines.

Clarity refers to content and writing that are easily understood. Terminology must be specific and meaningful to all members of the health care team. Abbreviations and symbols are avoided. Grammar and spelling are appropriate to the English language, and handwriting must be legible. Headings of the components and their subdivisions should be underlined.

Completeness refers to totality in content and sentence structure. Content is complete when all seven components are present; all necessary data are included in each component; and there are no doubts that certain questions were asked. Complete sentences, rather than phrases—telescopic language—are used to record the data, and contractions are avoided.

Conciseness means that the history is briefly stated yet complete. Completeness should never be sacrificed for conciseness.

Consecutiveness is the final characteristic. Data must be presented logically, and each component and its subsequent parts must follow in sequence.

Each of the five "c's" is applied in recording every component of the history. Their application will be emphasized in Part Two.

All records are dated, and require the signature and title of the person collecting the data.

PART II

COMPONENTS of
THE HEALTH HISTORY

CHAPTER **4**

REASON for CONTACT

The first part of this book discussed the components of the Health History and the methods of data collection and recording. As the components of the Health History are discussed in detail, keep in mind that those concepts and principles apply to each of the components.

The first component of the Health History is concerned with the basis, the motivation, or the underlying cause which has directed the client to the health care personnel and facility—*The Reason for Contact*. Appropriate questions which may be asked to elicit such information are: "What has brought you to the clinic, hospital or other health care facility?" or "What seems to be the problem?"

The Reason for Contact is a brief statement, in the client's (or informant's) own words, as to why he has come to the health personnel and facility. It would be recorded as follows:

> *Reason for Contact:* The client requested a "complete physical examination."

The *Reason for Contact* may be promotion of health, prevention of illness, or the maintenance and restoration of health.

In the past, and frequently still, the primary motivating factor for contacting health personnel was for illness—and the person contacted was the doctor. Today, an individual encounters a number of health personnel and facilities, and for a variety of purposes which may be either self motivated or encouraged by others. The client, in most instances, has definite expectations and feels the need for specific services.

For example, a person seeks health care as a requirement for employment. Since not all health problems are visible, the employer requests the examination for the purpose of uncovering major physical or emotional problems that might undermine the person's ability to meet the demands of the position. If this were not done, the employer would bear the expense of training or educating the employee at considerable cost, only to find the person nonproductive because of illness. The client might fear detection of an illness that would jeopardize his employment opportunities, or that an illness he has been hiding or coping with may be revealed. Even if he was successful and productive in previous jobs, the employer may regard the problem as too great a risk, and not hire him.

The "annual physical" has become increasingly popular both to fulfill a requirement for continued employment or promotion, and to meet the individual's desire for well-being. Most people are better informed today through mass media, and appreciate that early detection and treatment of illness may add years to life and productivity. Client concerns can best be appreciated by comments often made following the annual physical examination: "I just received a clean bill of health." "The doctor told me I am as fit as a fiddle." "Well, I am safe for another year." These all express relief that disease was not detected which would require a modification of life style for even a short period of time. A man who is very athletic and prides himself on his physical fitness may have his fears allayed by understanding that the stiffness he feels on getting out of bed in the morning is simply the result of too much physical activity the previous week, and not arthritis.

Similarly, the *Reason for Contact* may be to meet a request for a "school physical," and would be recorded in much the same way.

Reason for Contact: "I need a school physical."

In this instance, the importance of the contact may not always be fully appreciated. The client is young and sees himself as being healthy. He may look upon the "school physical" as an inconvenience—a form that needs to be filled out before he can attend school. Rarely (unless he has had specific education) does he view the experience as a means of promoting health or as protecting others from contagious diseases which he may carry. The young adolescent in particular may be upset and embarrassed by the whole thing—he knows that the "school physical" means having to undress. He may be at an age when he is self-conscious of his bodily changes, and the "physical" is a threat to his privacy.

Others may seek the services of health personnel and facilities for reasons such as family planning or family and genetic counseling. The *Reason for Contact* would simply be recorded as:

Reason for Contact: Client requests "advice about birth control."

or . . .

Reason for Contact: Client states that he has sickle cell anemia and questions how this will affect his child.

In the latter example the concern is related not to a personal illness, but to status as a carrier of a genetic trait that could affect offspring. Although his motivation is prevention of illness to someone other than himself, he is still quite anxious. He wants assurance that all is well—that his children will be normal at birth—but at the same time, he fears he will be told just the opposite.

However, not everyone who seeks preventive health care feels the same anxiety. A mother brings her son, Christopher, to a well-baby clinic for poliomyelitis immunization. She is following a prescribed routine for her son's health care. She knows that if Chris gets the vaccine, his chances of contracting polio are greatly diminished. She has no anxiety or fear because she is doing something specific to keep another individual free from disease. In this instance, the mother is the informant and the *Reason for Contact* would include this information:

Reason for Contact: Mother states "Chris is due for his polio vaccine."

Even today with more and more emphasis being placed on promotion of health and prevention of illness, you will find that the most common *Reason for Contact* is still illness or thoughts of illness. Seeking health care for "illness" may be thought of as maintenance or restoration of health. If there is a specific complaint regarding illness, then the *Reason for Contact* should be recorded as a brief statement in the client's own words which includes the symptoms and their duration and location. A symptom is any event that the client perceives as being a deviation from his normal state of health. It could relate to alterations in function, sensation, or appearance. Regardless of how the client describes his symptoms, you should avoid rephrasing his statement, and the use of diagnostic terms and names of diseases.

Let us say that in response to the question, "What seems to be the problem?" the client says, "It's my leg." Would this be a correct statement to record as the client's *Reason for Contact?* Your first response might be "Yes," for it is a brief statement in the client's own words. But, what is it about the client's leg that has motivated him to seek health care? Which leg is involved? How long have the symptoms been present? These are additional questions that will have to be asked in order to collect data as to the specific complaint—the *Reason for Contact.*

Assume that the client's response to your question is:

"For the past two weeks I haven't felt well."

You know the duration, but what does "I haven't felt well" mean? You might ask the client, "Can you tell me more specifically how you feel?" or "What do you mean?" In both instances, you must be careful that you do not create a situation where you are suggesting specific symptoms and turning the *Reason for Contact* into a statement in *your* words. This can happen, if instead of asking the question, "What is it about your leg that bothers you?" you say, "Do you have pain?" The client may answer "Yes" because he has a toothache which is causing pain. But you have no way of knowing that and you relate the pain to his leg. However, the real reason that the patient is seeking health care is for the rash he has on his leg and not the pain in his tooth.

You may also be tempted to help the client who does not "feel well" by identifying his symptoms and asking questions such as: "Do you have dyspnea?" "Do you ever have indigestion?" "Have you experienced difficulty urinating?" "Have you had insomnia?" He may not know the meaning of the terms, yet will answer "Yes" to all of your questions—still you do not know his specific complaint. What you have is a list of symptoms which you have given the client and which may or may not be related to the problem.

Too, you may find yourself in a very different situation. In response to your question, "What seems to be the problem?" Mrs. Miller begins:

Five years ago I was carrying my two year old son who has cerebral palsy, when suddenly I had a sharp pain in my back. I went to the doctor and he put me in the hospital because I had a slipped disc. I didn't seem to get any better, so he operated and made that part of my back stiff. I was fine, never had any problem—did everything—swimming, dancing, housework—everything. About a week ago, when I was food shopping I bent down to pick up a can of tomatoes and I felt a sharp pain in my back. I went home, took some aspirin and stayed in bed for two days. I felt better but the pain never really went away—but this morning when I got out of bed to see why the baby was crying—she had measles—I felt the sharp pain again. It is in my back, goes into the back of my hip and then down my right leg. I took some aspirin but my leg still hurts and my husband said . . . . on and on and on.

The verbose person can be very disconcerting. Not only has Mrs. Miller upset your orderly sequence of questions and provided you with information related to several components of the Health History, but she has left you with the problem of how to record her *Reason for Contact*. You might consider this:

> *Reason for Contact:* Five years post spinal surgery for herniated nucleus pulposus. One week ago, experienced recurrent pain, was relieved by bed rest and aspirin. Today, pain reappeared in lower back with sciatic pain radiating down her right leg.

Obviously, the above recording is incorrect. It is not a brief statement in the client's own words, and although it does identify symptoms, they have been rephrased and stated in diagnostic terms with the names of specific diseases. Also included are statements related to *Current Health Status* and *Past Health History*.

In this situation, the correct recording of the *Reason for Contact* would be:

> *Reason for Contact:* "I have pain in my back, the back of my hip and down my right leg, which began this morning."

That statement tells specifically why the client came to the health care facility that day. The remainder of the information can be jotted down, and elaborated upon under the appropriate components of the Health History. It is important, and should not be disregarded—it is all part of the Health History.

Summary

There are many reasons why an individual may seek the services of a variety of health care personnel and facilities—promotion of health, prevention of illness, or maintenance and restoration of health. As the individual becomes more sophisticated, his reason for selecting particular health care personnel or a specific facility may change. Nevertheless, the definition of the *Reason for Contact* will continue to be a brief statement in the client's own words as to why he has come. When illness is involved, the "why" will relate to specific symptoms and will include the duration and location of such symptoms. This information is always to be stated in the client's own words and not rephrased; nor does it utilize diagnostic terms and names of diseases unless he has used such terms.

chapter 5

biogRAphicAl dATA

Biographical Data are general sorts of information about "who" the client is and his background. They provide the starting point toward seeing the client as a total person, giving direction to and influencing the interview. These data may also be a significant factor in determining the client's health status.

Included in the *Biographical Data* are the client's "vital statistics": his full name and address; telephone number; age; date and place of birth; sex; ethnic group; religion; primary spoken language; marital, educational, and occupational status; health insurance and Social Security number. The parents' first names and mother's maiden name are further sources for identification.

You may question why you initially need this information, and why it would not be considered in the client's *Current Health Status* or *Past Health History*, if it is a significant factor in determining the client's health status. How can "vital statistics" direct or influence the interview?

The client's "vital statistics" serve as specific identifying data. This is of utmost importance since in some communities there may be more than one person with the same name—perhaps even with a similar address and age. Therefore, in collecting *Biographical Data* you will need to identify the client by his full name and address—John George Jones, 100 West 20th Street, New York, New York, 10012—not John G. Jones, 100 West 20th Street, N.Y., N.Y. John G. could mean John Gerald, John Gene, or John Gregory, who could be related to the client and live at the same address.

It is important to have the client's telephone number, including the area code; should you need to contact the client or his family, this will facilitate matters.

You might ask, "If you know the client's age, why do you need the date and place of birth?" The date of birth will verify the age. A discrepancy may give you additional data. (Is the client trying to hide his age? Does he have a memory deficit?) The place of birth may identify social or cultural factors that can relate to disease or indicate a language barrier. For instance, John George Jones, 33 years of age, presents at the clinic with complaints of multiple skin lesions on his cheeks associated with decreased sensation. The client also tells you he was born, and has lived on the Island of Molokai, until a few months ago. These facts could suggest that he may have leprosy.

The client's sex may not always be obvious; or he could have the physical appearance of one sex and yet identify himself with the other. Since certain conditions have a sexual predominance, this information is significant. Hemophilia, for example, is transmitted by females but appears exclusively in males. Such information also may help to identify aspects of psychosocial development that can affect the individual's well-being.

The client's ethnic background may have a bearing on his socialization process, food preferences, attitudes, and behaviors. It can also be directly related to certain disease processes. Example: A child of Jewish parentage arrives at the clinic. You learn that he is blind and is subject to convulsive seizures. The mother states that the child has regressed both mentally and physically. You consider the possibility of Tay-Sachs disease, which affects only Jewish persons.

Not all clients will share their religious beliefs; their right to privacy must be respected. However, such information is extremely useful in regard to care, especially of the hospitalized client. The chaplain, as a member of the health team, may play an important role in working with a client and family in crisis. An acutely ill client who is Roman Catholic may require the Sacrament of the Sick; a Jewish client may require a Kosher diet. Organizations with religious affiliations may offer aid to clients or families in need, by giving financial assistance or emotional support, or by making possible long-term or convalescent services.

The primary spoken language will influence the interview. It is frequently taken for granted that because the client has learned to speak English as a second language, he understands all the English that is spoken to him. If he does not fully understand your questions he may answer "Yes" to all of them, and thereby negate the whole point of the interview. To diminish frustration for both the client and yourself, you might want to seek help of an interpreter before you get into the details of data collection. Also, consider that a client experiencing stress may revert to his primary language, which could mislead others to believe that he does not speak or understand English.

Under Marital Status, identify whether the client is single, married, divorced, or widowed. (These relationships will be discussed under *Family History*.)

Knowing the client's educational background may enable you to direct your questions, during the remainder of the interview, to his level of understanding, or later to develop a specific teaching plan geared to his level of comprehension. Bear in mind that the level of education and of understanding may not correspond: you can assume that a client who has a college degree would have little, if any, difficulty answering your questions, in comparison to one who has a sixth-grade education; yet the one with the sixth-grade education may be self-educated, and his level of comprehension may be comparable to that of the college graduate. Identification of this fact will protect the client from insult and save you embarrassment. Talking down may "turn him off" and ultimately result in an incomplete Health History or a wrong evaluation of angry and hostile behavior. By the same token, using unfamiliar terms may frustrate or embarrass a person who does not understand them.

Knowledge of the client's occupation gives insight into his source of income, degree of self-esteem, and possibly to diseases to which he may be susceptible. His description of his occupation gives valuable clues as to how he sees himself. With great pride, he may say, "I am a bank teller." Or he may say, "I am just a bank teller." In the latter case, the clue he holds himself in low esteem may, indeed, indicate that this is affecting his health status, and warrants further investigation. Numerous diseases are directly related to occupation, so it is essential that occupation be identified. Also, a client may state that she is a housewife. What does this mean? Is she a full-time homemaker? A part-time one? A full-time housewife who employs a live-in maid and a cook certainly has a very different life from a full-time housewife who has six children, and lives on a farm which she helps to run.

Information regarding health insurance may be needed to aid the client to plan for hospitalization or to pay for laboratory tests, x-ray examination, clinic visits, medications, or visiting nurse services. Clients are sometimes reluctant to have tests done or to seek further health care because they are not aware of the extent of their health insurance and do not feel they can afford the prescribed care.

The Social Security number is a further means of identifying the client. The first names of both parents and the mother's maiden name also are recorded.

Biographical Data can be recorded in outline form when a standardized or a stamped form is supplied by the health care facility. For example:

Biographical Data

Name:	John George Jones
Address:	100 West 20th Street
	New York, New York, 10012
Telephone Number:	212-123-4567
Age:	33
Date & Place of Birth:	September 29, 1942
	Molokai, Hawaii
Sex:	Male
Ethnic Group:	Portuguese–Hawaiian
Religion:	Withheld
Primary Language Spoken:	English
Marital Status:	Divorced
Education Status:	High School
Occupation:	Unemployed 2 years
Health Insurance:	None
Social Security:	022-01-0033
Parents' Names:	John Jones; Mary Casey Jones

The above recording is concise and clearly stated; specific data are easy to identify. When a standardized form is not supplied by the facility, the *Biographical Data* are recorded in complete sentences and paragraph form, yet still are concise, clear, and easy to identify:

Biographical Data: Mr. John George Jones lives at 100 West 20th Street, New York, New York 10012; his telephone number is: 212-123-4567; and Social Security number is: 022-01-0033. He is 33 years old, divorced, English speaking male, born on the Island of Molokai, Hawaii, on September 29, 1942, and is of Portuguese-Hawaiian background. Mr. Jones, a high school graduate, has been unemployed for the past two years and is without health insurance. His primary spoken language is English and he has withheld his religious preference. His parents are John Jones and Mary Casey Jones.

Summary

The *Biographical Data* begins to introduce the client as a total person, as the *Review of Systems* serves as an overall check that all relevant data have been obtained. The data collected may influence the client's health status as they provide information which gives direction to or affects the interview. These include client's full name; address; phone number; age, date, and place of birth; marital, educational, and occupational status; health insurance; and Social Security number. The first names of parents and mother's maiden name are included. The *Biographical Data* may be recorded in outline form, when a standardized form is used, or in complete sentences in a brief paragraph.

CHAPTER **6**

CURRENT HEALTH STATUS

The *Current Health Status* provides a general impression of the client's present state of health. It includes details of the specific complaints if appropriate to the Health History, and the client's daily habits or activity patterns: diet; elimination; personal hygiene; use of tobacco and drugs; recreation and exercise; and sleep. It also may yield insight into the client's perception of his health. Therefore, this component will enable you to continue to identify not only "who" the client is, but "where" he is in terms of health: Are his specific complaints related to his daily activity patterns? Are his daily activities conducive to his growth and development? Are his activities in conflict with his health? Often, teaching or therapeutic advice takes into account data related to the client's activity patterns; this information is needed so that any necessary modification of behavior can be discussed with him.

Both specific complaints and daily habits are integral parts of the *Current Health Status.* If, however, the client is seeking health care because of a specific problem, this should then be dealt with accordingly. Delay in such questioning or failure to take appropriate action can communicate lack of sensitivity to his needs and contribute to his frustration and discomfort.

Specific Complaint(s)

Data collection for a specific complaint include: date and time of onset; characteristics of the complaint, location, length of time, quality; associated symptoms; effects on activities and body functions; cause of complaint if known; treatment received (where, by whom given, and its effect). This helps you to determine the acuteness of the complaint and to intervene appropriately. The following examples illustrate several approaches:

Example 1
Specific Complaint: At one a.m. Mrs. Pepper was awakened by severe abdominal cramps and vaginal bleeding. For the past five hours she has had "heavy vaginal bleeding." She says she has soaked ten large bath towels and passed six large clots "the size of a lemon." The cramps have gotten worse—"like a knife in my stomach that keeps stabbing." She says she feels very weak, cannot hold up her head, and fainted when she tried to walk.

In the case of Mrs. Pepper, who is acutely ill, you would interrupt the Health History immediately and provide care.

Example 2
Specific Complaint: Mrs. Lang states that Emily was awakened at two a.m. by a "sharp pain on her left side that radiated to her back." She described the pain as being "knife-like" and constant. The pain is less intense when she is lying on her left side with her knees drawn up. Mrs. Lang reports that Emily has vomited three times in the past two hours and feels very warm. Prior to retiring she complained of "feeling funny and hot," and was given two aspirin. Yesterday, Emily also complained of "burning when she urinated." Mrs. Lang says this often happens following her menstrual periods. Emily began menstruating six months ago. Her mother says her periods are regular, every twenty-eight days, bleeding is minimal and she does not complain of cramps. She has not been treated for the "burning when urinating" following her periods. Her last menstrual period was two weeks ago.

Emily also needs immediate care. However, she can be made more comfortable by being positioned on her left side with her knees flexed. Additional data can be collected from her mother, which may be helpful in further identifying her problem.

Example 3

Specific Complaint: Yesterday evening Mr. Jackson was playing baseball. He "fell into third base" and twisted his right ankle. Initially he did not have any severe pain, but could not put much weight on his foot. At ten p.m., the nature of the pain changed to intense, dull and throbbing. He says his right ankle was "two times the size of the left." He could not walk and had to lean on his friends to get to the hospital. In the emergency room, the right foot was x-rayed, an Ace bandage was applied, and he was instructed not to put any weight on his foot and was medicated for pain. This morning, upon awakening, he noticed his foot was "crooked and toes swollen and blue." The pain has increased . . . "it feels like there's a lot of pressure and the pills never worked." He says that he did not sleep well, "just couldn't get comfortable." He tried elevating his leg on two pillows and that "felt better."

In Mr. Jackson's case, you could complete the Health History after first elevating his leg and loosening the Ace bandage to decrease the discomfort.

As you continue to collect data related to the Current Health Status, you notice that the specific complaints particularly relate to the client's activity pattern, and that the problem is more complicated than it initially appeared. Consequently, your perception of the complaint changes. For instance, in Emily's situation, you might learn that her fluid intake is very minimal and her personal hygiene poor. Emily may have a chronic kidney infection. In Mr. Jackson's case, you may learn that he is an alcoholic, a factor which may be related to his injury and the ineffectiveness of the medication he was given.

If the *Reason for Contact* does not relate to a specific complaint, you might consider data about his reasons for seeking health care. For instance, if the client states his *Reason for Contact* is an "annual physical," you would ask him if there is anything bothering him now that made him decide it was time for an annual physical. You could record this in an opening praragraph:

Mr. Herrera has come to the clinic for an annual physical. He states he feels "fine," does not think there is anything wrong with him, but "always has an annual examination to be sure."

Daily Habits or Activity Patterns

Daily habits or activity patterns, as previously described, strongly influence one's health. Certain patterns often are so well established that the person is hardly aware of them. Consequently he may not fully appreciate the need for accuracy, and you may find it necessary to explain why such questions are required.

Diet

The assessment of dietary patterns, another important aspect of the client's health status, can be divided into three parts:

1. Factors related to recent weight gain or weight loss, including minimal and maximal weight and the respective age at which each was reached; present weight and height; and the client's ideas about weight.

2. Daily food intake. Regardless of whether the client chooses his daily food intake or follows a prescribed diet because of a specific problem, the assessment includes the types and amounts of food; cultural restrictions or preferences; frequency of meals; types and amounts of snacks; time of day when he feels most hungry; allergy or food intolerance; fad diets or supervised restricted intake; and environmental and economic problems.

3. Fluid intake, including frequency and amount of water, milk, soup, fruit juice, and alcoholic and caffeine beverages.

All of the above information should be viewed in relation to age, since nutritional needs change throughout growth and development. Environmental factors also may influence dietary patterns. Your purpose in collecting dietary data is to evaluate the suitability of diet to age and activity. By asking him to describe his food intake for a 24-hour period, you will be able to determine if he is getting the proper amounts of proteins, vitamins, minerals, fats, and carbohydrates. You then correlate these with the physical findings of height and weight; condition of skin and teeth; laboratory studies; and behavioral problems. Should you discover a specific nutritional deficit, you would note a need for education and supervision by a member of the health team; the deficit might be intimately related to the chief complaint.

Why include data on fluid intake? How can these affect the *Current Health Status?* Does it matter what or how much the client drinks? What does this information tell you?

Previously, you have learned that fluid helps regulate body temperature; transport various substances throughout the body; transport waste products to the kidney whence they are excreted in water; provide bulk within the intestinal tract to aid in elimination; and function in growth and repair of body tissue.

Infant needs for fluids are three times greater than the adult's, because water is much more abundant in the infant's body. The normal infant requires approximately 125 cc of fluid per kg of body weight per day; the normal adult, approximately 2500 to 3000 cc per day. Either inadequate or excessive fluid intake, or a sudden change in intake may be significant. A recently acquired thirst may be an early sign of diabetes mellitus; whereas in hot, humid weather it may serve as a protective response to excessive fluid loss through perspiration.

You can better evaluate the client's total fluid intake if you know not only what he drinks but also how much.

The following examples demonstrate both normal practices and those that necessitate client instruction.

Example 1

Diet: Mrs. Brown is five feet four inches tall; her weight has fluctuated between 120 and 130 pounds for the past 40 years; present weight is 125 pounds. She feels her weight is "just right—not too fat, not too thin." Her daily food intake consists of two cups of tea for breakfast; cheese, meat, fish, or eggs, salad, fruit, and one cup of tea for lunch; and meat, fish, or poultry, green vegetable, potato or bread, fresh fruit and one cup of tea for dinner. She usually has "a cup of tea and something sweet" midday. She drinks approximately six glasses of water per day. She reports no allergies or intolerance to foods, no cultural or religious restrictions on her diet. She does not like milk and she has never felt the need to diet. She cooks her own meals and usually eats at home alone. Occasionally she has a friend in for dinner but rarely goes out. "Every once in a while I just don't feel like cooking in the evening, so I may then just have a cup of tea."

Your initial assessment may be that Mrs. Brown's diet is adequate except for calcium, and that she has maintained a consistent weight for a long period of time which is appropriate for her height—but she is not eating breakfast, which nutritionists believe is a very important meal. Initially you may see this as a problem and feel that she needs instruction—but are you really going to change a dietary pattern that has existed for 40 years? Is it necessary? Since for her this is an adequate diet, the answer to both questions is no.

Example 2

Diet: Mr. Sanchez is 5 feet 6 inches tall and presently weighs two hundred pounds. He reports his weight was 160 pounds at age sixteen, following a supervised diet, and his weight was 210 pounds at age thirty-five, one year ago. Over the past ten years he has followed multiple fad diets, with his weight fluctuating from 175 to 210 pounds. Mr. Sanchez eats many times a day. He complains of hunger around eleven in the morning and four in the afternoon. Breakfast consists of a glass of juice, two cups of coffee and something sweet—"I crave sweets in the morning"; a cup of coffee and sweets at eleven; lunch is usually a meat sandwich, cake and two glasses of milk; candy at about four; a dinner of meat, vegetables, potatoes, bread, dessert and two cups of coffee. He then usually has cake or fruit and a glass of milk before bed. Mr. Sanchez rarely drinks water, but has a "couple of beers" with friends after work. He is allergic to strawberries but tolerates all other foods without difficulty. He says that he likes all foods and has no ethnic preferences. He lives alone, does not like to cook frequently—therefore, eats out with friends "maybe four or five times a week." He does not see himself as being overweight and says that eating gives him something to do and a chance to be with friends.

It is obvious that Mr. Sanchez has a dietary problem which could affect his health, and which will require specific health education, possibly including consultation with the nutritionist. His adherence to fad diets and his weight fluctuations are unhealthy. His carbohydrate intake is excessive; nevertheless his age suggests that it will be possible to bring about a change in his dietary patterns.

Example 3

Diet: Mrs. Hibbing reports that David is 36 inches tall and weighs 31 pounds, and that progression in height and weight during the first two years of his life has been "normal according to Dr. Spock." Until recently David has enjoyed his meal time, eating cereal, fruit and milk for breakfast; meat, eggs or cheese, a vegetable, bread and butter, gelatin and milk for lunch, a snack of milk and cookies following nap time; and meat, fish or poultry, a vegetable, milk and fruit for dinner. He drinks approximately three glasses of water during the day. For the past four weeks, David has refused to eat. Mrs. Hibbing tries to force him, and "he just spits out his food and says, 'No!'" to both the introduction of new foods and his favorite foods. Meal time for David has become very tense—"a major production." She has resorted to allowing David to snack on whatever he likes because she is afraid he will get sick.

Toddlers need an adequate diet to ensure tissue replacement needed for normal growth and development. Brief periods when they refuse to eat are to be expected; forcing food can lead to serious eating problems. David is of ideal height and weight for his age. In this instance, Mrs. Hibbing does not need specific dietary instruction about her two year old son, but does need help in understanding that David is experiencing a normal dietary pattern for his age.

Example 4

Diet: Judy, who is five feet five inches tall, weighs 90 pounds. Mrs. C. says that Judy progressed normally through growth and development in both height and weight and at age 14 she weighed 145 pounds. Three months ago Judy weighed 120 pounds. She has suddenly stopped eating, even though well-balanced meals containing meat, fish, eggs, vegetables, milk, and fruits are attractively prepared for her. Judy says she likes most foods, but she is on a diet because she is "too fat." She does not understand why she has to eat all "those foods" that her sister and mother will not eat. She sees nothing wrong with what she is doing and there is "so much commotion" around meal time, that she just does not want to be involved.

It would not be appropriate at this time to collect data relating to frequency of meals, preference for ethnic foods, allergies, etc. Although Judy is exhibiting fairly typical adolescent behavior, she is also endangering her health. Her refusal to eat goes beyond the fad diet phase, which so many adolescents experience; and she is past the stage of imitating parents or siblings who might influence her food preferences. She is markedly underweight for her height. Factors known to affect appetite negatively include unattractive foods or surroundings, and unpleasant company. Judy is offered attractively prepared foods yet describes meal time as a "commotion." Judy and her parents may need counseling. Or, should it be determined that Judy has anorexia nervosa, immediate medical care may be required.

Example 5
Diet: Jill weighed 8 pounds and was 21 inches long at birth. During the past three weeks, she has gained 12 ounces. She "eagerly drinks her bottle" of 3½ ounces of Similac formula, five times a day. On hot days her mother gives her an additional ounce or two of water. Jill burps readily and does not spit up.

Here is an illustration of the relationship between fluid, diet, and age. Young infants are maintained on a fluid diet, and Similac is one of the widely used liquid preparations that are prescribed. The volume of formula is appropriate to Jill's weight; and her mother's responses indicate that she understands that fluids are rapidly lost in hot weather and must be replaced. Therefore, the information communicates that Jill's intake is normal for her age, her weight gain is appropriate, and she is tolerating her diet well. No intervention is necessary at this time. You may wish to assure the mother that her actions are appropriate.

These examples illustrate how data related to weight, height, food and fluid intake, and growth and development can be integrated into the assessment of dietary patterns, from which a need for specific health care may be directed.

Elimination

Elimination is the next area to be assessed, since it is closely related to dietary intake. The color, frequency, characteristics, and odor of urine and feces are noted. Sudden or recent changes in bowel or bladder habits are included, since these may bear upon specific diseases. Any problem must be evaluated to determine whether it is truly related to elimination or results from the client's notions about "normal" elimination patterns. Note should also be made about any treatment the client may have had.

A young mother may tell you that she is concerned about her infant's health because his bowel movements are unlike those of her first child. She may state that the infant has several soft, rather spongy stools daily, which occasionally contain mucus, whereas her first child had only two stools daily which were yellow and more solid. Thus, you need to obtain data related to the child's feedings. The stool is normal for a breast-fed infant; the sibling's stool is normal for a bottle-fed infant.

Another mother may voice concern over her child's constipation. Since not every person has a daily bowel movement, you must first find out what the mother means by "constipation." Is it that her child does not have a daily bowel movement, or that the child goes for a period of five to six days without having a bowel movement? In the latter case, you may be able to discern from what she has already told you about the child's dietary pattern that his diet lacks bulk and that dietary instruction is called for. On the other hand, the problem could be related to the child's toilet training rather than to his diet; his constipation could have an emotional basis stemming from early toilet training. In any event, you need to have information concerning the mother's treatment of the constipation and the length of such treatment. If she is giving the child harsh laxatives or daily enemas, these can be extremely irritating to the bowel, contributing to loss of normal bowel function and electrolyte depletion. Then other body systems would also be involved, and this would influence the *Reason for Contact.*

Many adults also believe they should have a daily bowel movement, when in fact a bowel movement every three days may be normal for them. They, too, may resort to using laxatives or enemas, with similar effects. Determine when the constipation began. If the use of laxatives and enemas has become an established pattern, it may be necessary to educate the client about the significance of this dependency. The elderly person may have to continue this practice, since he is now dependent on laxatives or enemas. If marked changes in elimination are a recent occurrence, a bowel obstruction or lead poisoning could be the cause. Any change demands further study.

A complaint of diarrhea is associated with other problems. Frequent episodes may be related to factors in the environment which cause stress. Questioning along these lines may help to further identify the cause.

In an infant, the diarrhea may be due to an indigestible formula. Since infants quickly become dehydrated—a serious problem—you need to learn how long the problem has been present. An adult may tell you that his diarrhea began three weeeks ago, and may definitely relate the onset to drinking water in Mexico. Adults, too, can become dehydrated and may require immediate care.

Other types of bowel elimination may be correlated with specific pathology. In the infant, a bloody stool of currant-jelly consistency, followed by sudden cessation of bowel movements, may indicate intussusception. In the young adult, small stools containing mucus, blood, or pus associated with occasional diarrhea may point to ulcerative colitis. A fecal impaction may be diagnosed on the basis of complaints of a combination of constipation and watery diarrhea.

The record of elimination may be quite detailed. Referring back to Mrs. Hibbing's situation:

> *Elimination:* Mrs. Hibbing also reports that prior to David's lack of interest in eating, he had had a daily bowel movement, which was well formed, brown, and soft. Now his bowel movements are about every four days apart, brown, and very hard. Since David has not complained, she has not instituted treatment.

In contrast, Mr. Sanchez, who is overeating, may tell you:

> *Elimination:* "I've been constipated for the past six months." His normal bowel habits were daily stools, brown and well formed. He now finds that unless he takes "something," he does not have a bowel movement for four to five days, does have abdominal pain and with "straining" produces a hard dark brown stool with red streaks and rectal pain. He takes "Ex-lax," and when that is not effective will take an enema at night which relieves his constipation.

Difficulties with elimination may center around urine voiding; in this case fluid intake must be correlated with fluid output. The client may tell you that he drinks "large amounts" of fluid, yet his need to void is minimal. The frequent voiding of small amounts of urine or the voiding of cloudy urine may indicate a bladder infection; dark urine, concentration. A report of bright red urine may mean frank bleeding, and requires immediate evaluation. In children, dribbling needs to be distinguished from enuresis and from infection. Dribbling could be a sign of a structural anomaly in the child and the adult.

Bladder elimination should not be confused with bowel elimination. Questions related to both should be kept separate, but the data included in the same records. Thus, the second paragraph in David's elimination history might read:

> Mrs. Hibbing states that David's voiding pattern has not changed. She still needs to change him four times during the day and once at night. The color of his urine is "like straw" and the odor is that of "normal urine."

The second paragraph in Mr. Sanchez's elimination history may indicate further problems:

> For about two months his urine has been a very pale yellow and without odor. He voids "a lot—sometimes in very small amounts, other times in large amounts." He wakes up at least twice a night to urinate. He denies any other difficulties.

Personal Hygiene

Interviewing a client about his personal hygiene is very difficult simply because it is so intimate. Yet, such daily practices as proper care of mouth and teeth are necessary to the preservation of health. Because this is such a difficult subject to deal with, you may tend to deviate from the Health History and place a value judgment on what you see, confusing personal hygiene with appearance. Perhaps the most misjudged group in recent years has been the "hippies" with their "dirty long hair." There is nothing to say that a person with long hair is a hippy, or that long hair is invariably dirty. Value judgments are unfair and can be misleading; these are not recorded in the Health History.

Inherent to personal hygiene are factors such as bathing, hair washing, manicuring, and brushing teeth. Whether or not the client needs assistance with daily hygiene depends on his age and the extent of any disability that may exist. A child requires parental guidance and assistance which is influenced by the parents' view of the importance of personal hygiene. The client's culture, life style, and perception of hygiene will influence his routine. A teenage girl may feel the need to have shiny hair and may wash her hair daily; an elderly woman may feel frequent hair-washing causes her hair to fall out and washes her hair every two weeks. The "Saturday night bath" may be a part of the client's life style. If daily bathing was seen as important from infancy on, then this practice will probably continue. Living arrangements and socioeconomic factors also come into play. A client who lives in one room and shares a community bathroom facility may not bathe frequently.

Your questions must be carefully worded so that an accurate history will be obtained. A client who is asked if he takes a bath every day may say "No," thinking that you are referring to a tub bath; since only a shower is available, he does shower daily. A client who has dentures may not recognize that brushing one's teeth and cleaning one's dentures are essentially the same thing.

When you are interviewing a parent concerning a child's hygiene, it is helpful to know what types of assistance are offered to the child. Handing a two-year old a toothbrush and expecting him to brush his teeth without supervision is not likely to bring about effective tooth-cleaning. The child may just eat the toothpaste off the brush. A three-year old who is put into a tub to wash himself may become so engrossed in water play that he forgets to clean his ears and his neck.

Sample recording:

Personal Hygiene: Mr. Ruggles showers and washes his hair every morning and showers again every evening before retiring. He says that he bites his nails, so he "doesn't have to worry about that." He has a partial lower denture which he "soaks" every night, and he brushes his teeth, morning and night. He says that recently he had "bad breath" and now uses a mouth wash in the morning, once during the day, and again at night.

Tobacco and Drugs

The client may use substances that are potentially hazardous to his health or in the case of females, to the health of a fetus. Therefore, data related to length of use, amount and frequency of tobacco use (cigarettes, pipes, or cigars), sedatives, barbiturates, narcotics, amphetamines, laxatives, and alcohol are obtained. Not only drugs which might be considered abusive, but *all* drugs which the client may be taking—either prescribed by a doctor or self-prescribed, for example aspirin or cold tablets—should be recorded as part of the *Current Health Status.*

Collect as much information about the drugs as possible. The client may not be able to tell you the exact name of the prescribed medication, but may say, "a small pink pill for my heart," "I'm on the pill," or "I take a nerve pill." Reference may be made to medications by categories such as anticoagulants, antibiotics, antihypertensives, insulin. The client who can provide precise information leaves little room for guessing.

Data related to prescribed or self-administered drugs must be carefully evaluated as a reference point in future teaching. A woman who is pregnant may not appreciate that her drug habits can affect her unborn child. She may not realize that her addiction to narcotics can be transmitted to her child and that the child may be born an addict or that her excessive intake of alcohol may cause malformations in her child.

A client who is taking a prescribed drug which he categorizes as an "anticoagulant" may not be aware that with his self-prescribed drug, "aspirin," he may have a dangerous combination. The client who takes his antihypertensive drug only when he does not feel well may also be jeopardizing his health. A client might not be able to overcome an infection because he took his antibiotics for three days only, instead of the ten days prescribed. His responses will differ from those of the client who has taken the antibiotic for the ten days and still has the infection. One who "forgets" to take his insulin may also be denying the existence of his disease. Specific instruction may be needed to help him understand his illness; consultation with a specialist may be in order.

The *Current Health Status* should include a recording along these lines:

Tobacco and Drugs: Mr. Bisceglia has smoked cigarettes for the past twenty years. Until two years ago he smoked three packs per day but has cut back to six cigarettes per day, which he smokes following meals and in the evening when relaxing.

Mr. Bisceglia does not use sedatives, barbiturates, narcotics, amphetamines, or laxatives. "I don't like pills." He only takes them when prescribed and when he knows the reason. Mr. Bisceglia takes Coumadin, 5-10 mg, as prescribed by his doctor, at six pm daily. He says that he knows the drug keeps his "blood thin" and is "careful" about taking the medication, and knows that he should never take aspirin. He drinks socially—one or two scotches per week, usually during the weekend.

Recreation and Exercise

If a client does not appreciate the relationship of recreation and exercise to his health, he may regard exercise and recreation as completely separate entities, inasmuch as many recreational activities do not directly involve exercise. However, when the broad definition of health—physical, social, and mental well-being—is considered, their relevance becomes apparent. For a child, play is both recreation and exercise.

The adult needs diversional activities to refresh his mind and body. The old cliche "all work and no play makes Johnnie a dull boy" should have added to it, "and affects his general state of health." With never a break from daily pressures and a chance to relax, both physical and mental problems become more likely. Exercise assists in maintaining and building muscle strength and joint function; prevents deformity; stimulates circulation; and builds tolerance and endurance.

Children learn through playing: they develop motor skills; acquire control of their bodies; gain coordination; and begin to relate to people. Hence, when assessing play, one also assesses the child's activity tolerance. Does he engage in activities yet soon find himself on the sidelines watching the other children? Information relating to play habits will also enable you to better evaluate the child's growth and development.

Appropriate information in this section would include: amount, frequency, and type of recreation and exercise, whether on an individual or an organized basis; clubs; swimming, tennis, walking; reading; music; crafts.

Situation 1—Suzi, Age 2½
Mrs. Wong states that Suzi does not play with other children. When they are present, she "clings to me" and watches. She has a teddy bear that she carries with her at all times and she cries if another child attempts to take the toy. She ignores her kiddy car and is not a very active or inquisitive child—and she is very clumsy. Suzi is a quiet child, not like her brother who used to "empty my closets, scribble on the walls, pull his toys around, and do all those things even at a younger age." Suzi really "does nothing."

You might conclude that Suzi's play pattern is atypical for a child of her age. She should be doing things that require the use of her large muscles, and should be learning to play alongside another child. Further study is needed to determine her level of growth and development.

Situation 2—Jeffery, Age 7

Jeffery says he has "lots of hobbies" and the one he likes best is "collecting rocks." He plays outdoors with his friends, goes fishing twice a week and is very interested in sports, making puzzles and playing "inside games" with his friends on rainy days.

Jeffery's current play activities are consistent with his age.

Adult recordings are more detailed:

Situation 3—Mr. Green—Age 36

Mr. Green states his interests are many and varied. He enjoys sports activities and doing things with people. He swims twice a week and when the weather's good plays tennis every day. He also enjoys reading, which he finds relaxing, and refinishing furniture in his workshop. He vacations once a year with his family, usually camping and sight-seeing with the children. He does not belong to many groups—only the town council which meets four times a year.

Mr. Green's activities are consistent with his age and should support his health status. In contrast, there is Mr. Brittingham:

Situation 4—Mr. Brittingham—Age 50

Mr. Brittingham says that he is too tired to do anything but his work. Occasionally, he goes to the movies, but mostly he sits home and watches television. He says that there are many clubs in the neighborhood that he could join but "it's not the money." He is not interested and prefers to stay home. "Besides, I did all that once." He also states that he has not taken a vacation "that amounted to anything" in ten years.

Mr. Brittingham seems to be in a "rut." His lack of interest may be due to any number of factors—inability to form relationships, occupational demands, or previous health problems. Further investigation is needed to determine what has caused his attitude regarding group activities to change. His reasons may direct your attention to more detailed questioning in other parts of the Health History, such as the Family, Social, and Past Health Histories.

Sleep Patterns

Sleep is essential for maintenance of good health. All body processes slow down during sleep, and body tissues and organs are refreshed following the day's activities. The amount of sleep needed by each person varies according to constitution, activity, and age. Lack of sleep, or sleep deprivation for long periods of time, may give rise to irritability, memory loss, or hallucinations. It may also cause physical illness, since body tissues and organs do not have a chance to recuperate. Conversely, an individual may have episodes of falling asleep uncontrollably (narcolepsy) or may have encephalitis. Excessive sleep may be associated with boredom, a desire to escape unpleasant situations, strenuous physical activity, or with illness. Hence sleep patterns merit careful recording. The data to be collected are: the number of hours of sleep per night; quality of sleep; difficulty falling asleep; frequent interruptions in sleep (the number of times, causes); naps (length and time of day). As you are interviewing the client, keep in mind his age—there is a wide range of sleep patterns in various age groups.

One adult may have six hours of uninterrupted sleep every night and feel fully rested upon awakening; his sleep pattern is adequate for his needs. A mother may tell you that her newborn infant is sleeping only six hours a day. This would be a highly significant factor; during the first few months of life, an infant needs about 15 to 20 hours of sleep per day. If the adult who reports six hours of sleep describes his sleep as restless, his energy store may be low.

Difficulty in falling asleep affects various age groups in different ways. The adult client may be overtired; may have concerns, fears, or anxieties about his employment, family, and other responsibilities. The child, too, may have fears—the one- to two-year old fears his mother's leaving; the six-year old now has a concept of death. Other factors which interfere with the child's getting to sleep are: overstimulation at bed time; being put to bed and immediately being left in a dark room; a favorite toy or blanket that is missing; a noisy household; or simply a wet diaper. If a parent's complaint is the child's inability to get to sleep, then it would be helpful to ask such questions as: "What does your child do prior to bedtime?" "What is your routine in putting your child to bed?" "Is there a night light in the child's room?" "Does he sleep with a favorite toy?" One highly relevant factor that must be considered is whether the problem is the child's inability to get to sleep or the parent's inability to get the child to sleep. At times most children will resist—particularly toddlers, who are so interested in what they are doing they do not know they need sleep.

Frequent interruptions in sleep should be noted also. Adults may waken due to the need to empty the bladder, to nightmares, or to such normal reasons as the need to feed a newborn infant. The infant awakens when he has discomfort—usually hunger or pain; the three-year old because of frightening dreams—he has difficulty distinguishing the real from the imaginary; the six-year old may have nightmares concerning death, about which he now has some perception. Children of school age years may have enuresis which disrupts sleep. Is stress a factor? A small bladder? An organic lesion? Thus, when interviewing the client or the parent, ask "How frequently is sleep interrupted?"

The nap is common to all age groups and may have a cultural component. In many cultures, it is customary to rest following the midday meal. Adults, particularly the aged ones, may require a nap during the day. It is not unusual for a person who is depressed to use sleep as an escape.

Children have various nap patterns. The normal progression is from sleeping throughout most of the 24 hours, to having a morning and an afternoon nap, then to having one nap a day. At age four, nap time becomes a battle with the mother; the preschooler is so busy with what he is doing he does not know he needs sleep. The parent may be insisting on a nap regardless of age, misjudging the child's needs for rest; a consequence might be difficulty in getting the child to bed at night. Problems related to sleep must be discussed with the parent and assistance offered toward designing a plan for adequate and restful sleep.

The information to be collected includes the following: How frequently does the client nap? Has the frequency of naps changed? If so, when was this noted? Was it related to a particular set of circumstances? What time of day does he nap? For how long? Does he seem rested following a nap? In the case of a child, it might also be helpful to have the parent describe the child's behavior when he does not nap, as well as the effect on the parents' routine.

Sleep Patterns: Mr. Hoffman sleeps approximately six hours per night, which he feels is adequate to meet his needs. He does not have difficulty falling asleep; his sleep is not interrupted and he feels well rested upon awakening. Naps are not part of his daily routine, but he does nap following periods of strenuous activity such as a day of skiing.

Summary

The *Current Health Status* is the evaluation of the client's specific complaints, and of his daily habits or activity patterns. It contains details about these specific complaints; diet; elimination; personal hygiene; use of tobacco and drugs; recreation and exercise; and sleep. It provides a general impression of the client's present state of health and enables the practitioner to further identify not only "who" the client is, but "where" he is in terms of health. Since instruction or therapy may be based on data related to the specific complaints and daily habits or activity patterns, the relevance of this information can readily be appreciated.

pAST HEALTH HISTORY

The *Past Health History* relates information concerning the client's previous state of health or illness and contact with health care personnel and facilities. This includes previous developmental data, promotive and preventive practices, restorative intervention, allergies, and foreign travel. There are several reasons why these data have a place in the total assessment.

First, knowledge about the previous state of health will assist in assessing present problems, predicting responses, and planning immediate and long term care. If a 47-year old client who is admitted for a herniorrhaphy tells you that he has had no developmental problems, has "not been ill a day in my life," and that he has "a physical, including chest x-ray, and electrocardiogram every year," you will be less likely to expect any complications. Based on this information about positive health, you would plan routine preoperative teaching and anticipate that any discharge instruction for continuity of care would be followed.

Another reason is that in many illnesses there is an acute phase, followed by resolution, but with serious late consequences. Rheumatic fever, as an example, may cause valvular damage, yet no ill effects may be noted until, in adult life, such stresses as pregnancy or illness cause a flare-up.

Third, physical or mental limitations may result from illness or injury. Physical trauma as from an automobile accident may have necessitated a leg amputation, and the client may wear a prosthesis. A myocardial infarction may have necessitated restrictions in activity.

Finally, the presence of one disorder may cause heightened susceptibility to other diseases. A person who has diabetes mellitus, for instance, has an increased susceptibility to infection, yet, unless specific questions are put to him, he may not understand that they are important enough to be mentioned. A history of cancer, myocardial infarction, or ulcers, to cite just a few disorders, may provide a clue to causative factors in the event characteristic symptoms recur. Example: the client states that he had medical treatment for a duodenal ulcer three years ago. Last year the symptoms recurred, and part of his stomach was removed.

If it is readily verified that the past illness or injury is directly related to the *Reason for Contact,* the data are recorded under the *Current Health Status.* In the *Past Health History,* a notation would be made to refer the reader to the *Current Health Status* for details. Frequently, the relationship between the client's past and present state of health is not readily discerned. For example, the *Reason for Contact* may be, "Last night I felt short of breath." The *Past Health History* reveals that the client had had a myocardial infarction one year ago and a radical mastectomy three years ago. Further assessment would be necessary before the shortness of breath could be related to the possibility of either heart failure or metastasis.

Developmental Data

The developmental data include information specific to past physical, cognitive, and psychosocial parameters of development. These parameters for the client's present developmental period are included throughout all components of the Health History. Emphasis in the *Past Health History* is placed on any period in which there is indication that the client has had difficulties. The information serves as a guide in assessing current problems or in predicting those that might occur. A client may tell you that at the age of one year he was found to have a congenitally dislocated hip. He was treated with "a plaster cast, but it didn't help." He underwent numerous surgical procedures; although he cannot remember the dates, he says that he spent most of his time, from ages eight to 14, in the hospital. Finally, at age 14, his hip was fused, resulting in residual shortening of the leg and a "stiff hip." Hence you know not only that his past problem affected his ambulation, but also that the length of time he spent in the hospital during his childhood may have interfered with other aspects of development. He might not have been able to interact with other children, attend school, have close friends, or to gain a measure of independence. The lack of any of these could be the basis for psychosocial stress.

The stages to be included in the developmental history are: prenatal, paranatal, neonatal, infancy, toddler, early childhood, late childhood, adolescence, young adulthood, middle adulthood, and late adulthood. It is not within the scope of this book to present the specific characteristics of each of these stages of development. Some of the major areas to be assessed for each period will be delineated. The physical, cognitive, and psychosocial parameters should be considered in each stage. (See Chart 7-1.) In assessing the physical parameter, you should include a yearly height and weight record until young adulthood. After age 18 it is necessary only to record height and minimum and maximum weight. Recent changes in either height or weight are to be noted. Once maximum height is achieved, there probably will be no variation, until late adulthood when there may be some shortening due to skeletal changes. Gross motor movement—walking, jumping, catching a ball—is assessed, as are fine motor movements—thumb-finger pinch or grasp, writing, drawing, and building with blocks. To further assess the physical parameter, inquire about the client's

CHART 7-1. **Parameters for Each Stage of Development**

Physical
> General body growth
>> Height
>> Weight
> Muscular abilities
>> Gross motor movements
>> Fine motor movements
> Activities of daily living

Cognitive
> Intelligence
> Language
> Reasoning
> Concepts of nature, time, space, and causality
> Conceptual thinking

Psychosocial
> Personality
> Interactions with others
> Self-concept
> Recreation and play
> Roles
> Statuses

---

ability to perform activities of daily living—eating, bathing, dressing, elimination, exercise, and sleeping. These have a place in assessment at any age or stage of life.

The second parameter to be assessed for each stage is cognition, which encompasses intelligence; language; reasoning; concepts of nature, time, space, and causality; and conceptual thinking. Cognition is difficult to assess because the client does not have an accurate memory of early achievement in vocabulary or ability to count; nor can he recall early ideas about religion. An account given by an accompanying adult, or records of previous relevant examinations, will provide accurate information.

The third parameter is psychosocial development. Inquire about the client's personality, interaction with others, self-concept, recreation and play, roles, and statuses. Psychosocial tasks as presented by Erik H. Erikson can serve as a guide. These tasks will be discussed again briefly in relation to each state.

The *prenatal period* comprises conception to birth. Since the state of the mother's health and environment has a major effect on fetal development, questions should be raised about these. The mother is asked to describe her pregnancy. Key questions: Did the mother have medical supervision during the pregnancy? Was her diet nutritionally adequate? Did she experience any illnesses, infections, or complications? What drugs did she take? Were any treatments or procedures required? What was the duration of the pregnancy?

The *paranatal period* is the time of birth. Trauma during birth may cause serious disorders in the newborn, so you should obtain information about the course of labor and delivery, the type of delivery, the fetal presentation, and the methods of sedation and anesthesia. Record any complications.

The stage from birth through two to four weeks—the *neonatal* or *newborn period*—is one of the most stressful periods for the infant as he adjusts to the outside world. You want to inquire about the risk classification, the Apgar score, birth weight and length, congential anomalies, feeding, elimination, sleep patterns, length of hospital stay, and weight at discharge. The informant may not know what the Apgar score was, or may not understand the phrase (which is an evaluation of the newborn's heart rate, respiratory effort, muscle tone, reflex irritability, and color within 60 seconds after birth) and may be able to tell you only that "they said my baby was fine. He didn't have any trouble." If the exact score is unavailable, that is quite adequate for the assessment. During the neonatal period the main focus is on assessing the physical parameter. It is, however, during this time that the child is beginning to gain a sense of trust. To assess this, you should ask questions about the parents' reaction to the newborn, the time spent with him, and the reaction of siblings to his presence.

The next developmental stage to assess is *infancy,* the period from two to four weeks through one year of age. Record the infant's weight and height at six months and again at one year. Also record the age at which he sat, stood, crawled, walked, spoke, and was weaned, and the appearance of his first tooth. The infant's pattern of sleep and feeding or nursing should be included. Since the sense of trust is still an early stage of development, it is quite important to assess his reaction to separation, his social interactions, and the reactions of parents and siblings to him.

The *toddler period,* from one to three years of age, is characterized by increased mobility and a spirit of adventuresomeness and daring. The child is developing a sense of autonomy, of having some control over his activities. He is gaining control of speech, bodily functions, self-care, and interactions with others. There are rapid changes in the physical, cognitive, and psychosocial parameters during this period. Your questions center around the major tasks:

What was his yearly weight and height?
What assistance did he provide in feeding and bathing himself?
When was he bladder and bowel trained?
What interested him?
When did he start talking in phrases?
Did he have temper tantrums?
How well did he play with others?

During the *early childhood* or *preschool period,* from three to six years of age, the child needs independence, yet security at the same time. He is developing a sense of initiative, and wants to know what he can do and how far he can go. He is also learning many new words, developing new cognitive skills, and gaining greater motor skills. Although these years are referred to as "preschool," many children begin kindergarten or preschool at four or five years of age. The child's adjustment to the school situation should be elicited. Because there are rapid changes from year to year, it is best to focus questions upon those behaviors expected for the specific age rather than for the entire period. Some questions that will assist you in assessing the three developmental parameters:

At what age did he walk up and down stairs, dress and undress himself, go to toilet without assistance, and feed himself?
When did he begin to speak complete sentences?
Was he able to play games with others?
How far could he count when four years old?

Additional questions relative to other aspects of physical, cognitive, and psychosocial development such as sleep, weight, height, self-care, vocabulary, and personality should also be asked.

The child has gained many motor skills and is developing a sense of industry by the *later childhood* or *school age period,* from six to 12 years of age or puberty. He wants to do useful things and do them well. It is difficult to set norms for physical development during this period. You should, however, still note the yearly weight and height. You also need to inquire about the child's interactions with others, his play and school activities, self-care, sleep, and any employment such as newspaper route. Special hobbies and talents should be recorded.

The *adolescent period* spans the years from 12 to the beginning of adulthood—about 18 years of age. The adolescent is developing a sense of self-identity. There are rapid growth periods just prior to, or during, the first years of adolescence. Secondary sexual characteristics develop and, in girls, the onset of menses. You should include questions about these physical changes as well as the individual's reaction to them, for they can be significant psychosocial stressors. Next, inquire about the client's relationship with parents, siblings, friends and acquaintances, school, play, employment, and special interests. If career goals were established during this period, they should be recorded.

The years from 18 to 35 are considered the *young adulthood period.* It is during this stage that the vast majority of people develop a desire for intimacy by establishing a lasting relationship with a person of the opposite sex. The young adult is becoming creative, productive, and independent from his parents and beginning to establish his own home. He is pursuing a career choice.

The *middle adulthood period* covers the period from 35 to 65 years of age with the major task to establish and guide the young generation. As with other stages of development, there are changes from year to year or at least from the first years to the end of the period. During the first years, the tasks center around child rearing and work. There may be stresses if goals that the individual has set for either himself or others have not been met. This is a time for evaluation of one's life and reassessment of goals. Toward the end of the period, signs of aging begin to appear. The wrinkles, gray or sparse hair, failing vision, and physical illness may be a cause of concern about body image. Social changes impose social stress, as children marry and leave home to start families of their own. Retirement may now be considered. For some these are happy times, for others these are seen as the end of a productive life.

The *late adulthood* or *old age period* covers the years from 65 on. Then one assesses his own life and relationships with others. It is a time when one seeks to adapt to the successes and the disappointments of life. If the person is unable to feel that his was a life worth living, he may become deeply despondent. There may be increasing dependence upon others for care as a result of changes in the three parameters of development. Physical illness, decreased activity, loss of economic security, memory impairment, loss of family and friends, and loss of ability to care for self may play a role. Another task of the period is to prepare oneself to die. This most difficult task may be regarded as a release from a life no longer meaningful or as the end of a life well lived.

Promotive and Preventive Practices

Promotive and preventive practices include routine physical examinations, counseling services, and immunizations. This information serves as a guide to care planning; for example, education concerned with health practices. Question the client about partial or complete examinations, including routine physical, dental, ophthalmic, breast, chest, "Pap" test, and electrocardiograms. Their frequency and the date, place, significant results, and name of examiner should be recorded.

Notation is made about the use of counseling services, e.g. genetic, marriage, sex, planned parenthood, child guidance, and diet. A brief description of the situation necessitating the services and the results should be elicited.

To obtain data about the client's protection from or susceptibility to communicable diseases, information about the type and date of various immunizations is recorded. Those that are to be noted in the record include: diphtheria, tetanus, pertussis, poliomyelitis, mumps, measles, and tuberculin skin test. Note also should be made if they were not received. Others such as smallpox, yellow fever, and influenza ("flu") are included only if the client has received them. It is difficult for a client to remember whether or not he had the immunizations, much less the date or facility, so school records, armed services records, and foreign travel records may be useful in pinpointing dates. If the client has difficulty remembering, he might be encouraged to keep a record for all future immunizations.

A typical record of promotive and preventive practices:

Mr. Steinberg has a yearly physical examination, including electrocardiogram. The last examination, done by Dr. R. Jones, was on June 7, 1975. All findings were "normal." He has routine dental examinations by Dr. J. Brull, every six months. The last time was in September, 1975. His last eye examination was two years ago. He has an appointment with Dr. S. Owens for next month. He has had no counseling services. His examinations and immunizations were all done at the Neighborhood Health Center in Pelham, New York. His immunizations are:

1. Diphtheria, tetanus, pertussis and polio vaccine at two, four and six months of age and again when two and six years old;
2. Rubeola and tuberculin skin test at one year;
3. Mumps and rubella at six years;
4. Tetanus and diphtheria at sixteen and thirty years; and
5. Smallpox at age thirty.

Restorative Interventions

Review of any past illnesses, injuries, and surgery is listed under Restorative Interventions. Information about these conditions should be as complete as possible: date of occurrence, specific symptoms, cause if known, course of illness, treatment, complications, residual disability, and the health personnel and facility providing services. For example, if a client tells you only that he had pneumonia, you do not have much information. Did he have it one week ago or five years ago? Was he hospitalized? Did any complications develop? Did he have a high fever? What treatment was given? The following record provides you with the necessary information:

> In June, 1965, Mr. Grunsby had a high fever, chills, cough with "brownish" sputum, and pain on the right side of his chest. He was admitted by Dr. J. Brown for two weeks to Mt. Hope Hospital, Los Angeles, California, where he was diagnosed as having "pneumonia." He was treated for a "few days" with bed rest, penicillin, and oxygen. He returned to work two weeks following discharge and has had no recurrence.

Another client may say, "I had a nervous breakdown." If this is all that is recorded, you do not have much insight into the nature of the problem. What exactly does the client mean by "nervous breakdown"? What were his symptoms? Did he receive psychotherapy? Was he hospitalized? The following record is more complete:

> In December, 1974, Mr. Hilary was admitted to Psychiatric Institute, Detroit, Michigan, for two months because of severe melancholy, feelings of helplessness, and fatigue. He was diagnosed as being depressed and treated with "pills" and "psychotherapy," which he has continued until the present. He still becomes depressed at times, but he feels that these are the normal "ups and downs of life—not like the others." His therapist is Dr. Myron Smith.

Throughout the collection of the Health History, precise names of all medications should be obtained whenever possible. If this cannot be done at the initial interview, the client should be asked to bring in the bottles or vials so they can be identified.

Question the client about his experience with infectious diseases if these have not been included under the specific illnesses. Inquire about rheumatic fever, chickenpox, malaria, scarlet fever, diphtheria, pertussis, measles, mumps, poliomyelitis, and tuberculosis. The response is recorded with a description similar to that for other illnesses.

Allergies

Allergies, their manifestations, and the treatment thereof (including desensitization and medications), and the outcome of each are recorded. If the client has been tested for allergens, record the name of the tests and the results. Often the client does not know if he has an allergy; therefore, questions are to be asked about the presence of itching, skin lesions, fever, chills, sneezing, or wheezing when he is exposed to the chief allergens:

    1. Inhalants—pollens, fungi, dusts, vapors.

    2. Foods—wheat, eggs, milk, chocolate.

    3. Drugs and biologicals—penicillin, sulfonamides, phenothiazine, barbiturates, blood transfusions.

    4. Infectious agents—bacteria, fungi, parasites, viruses.

    5. Contactants—plastics, rubber, metal, chemicals.

    6. Physical agents—heat, cold, light, pressure.

All positive responses should be listed. Also, a notation should be made if the client has ever had penicillin or has had blood transfusions and whether he had an adverse reaction to either. The reason for this is so that health personnel can observe very closely for an adverse reaction the first time either penicillin is administered or blood transfusion is given. Here is one record:

> Mr. Goldman has had no allergies except for local skin redness under the metal portion of his watch. He has received antibiotics, including penicillin, without any reactions. He has not had a blood transfusion.

Foreign Travel

Foreign travel, other than that related to occupation, is recorded in the *Past Health History*. Since some conditions are endemic to certain countries or to certain sections of a country, it is necessary to know where the client has traveled. In this book, foreign travel refers to any area outside the normal habitat; for a client from Vermont, this would include travel to California, as well as to India or Germany. The client may not realize that there could be a relationship between his recent journeys and his current health problem, unless appropriate questions are asked. For example, a client may tell you that he was traveling throughout Southeast Asia during the summer. About two weeks after he returned, he experienced chills, fever, headache, and weakness; he thought he had "the flu." He became concerned, however, when a skin rash and lesions developed. Your knowledge about his recent travels focusses your attention on the possible diagnosis of smallpox. The notation in the record might be:

> Two weeks ago Mr. Edmunds returned from a three month vacation in Southeast Asia. He has not traveled to any other areas within the past years.

Summary

Information about the client's previous state of health or illness is elicited in the *Past Health History*. This information includes: developmental data—physical, cognitive, and psychosocial parameters—for the period in which difficulties are indicated; promotive and preventive practices—examinations, counseling, and immunizations; restorative interventions—past illnesses, injuries, and surgery; allergies; and foreign travel. A full description of promotive and preventive practices and restorative interventions should be presented. These data are important because they assist in predicting responses to therapy; many illnesses have an acute phase which subsides, but later is followed by serious sequelae; limitations may result from illnesses or injuries; and there can be an increased susceptibility to other conditions or recurrence of the same condition.

CHAPTER 8

family history

Before presenting the specific information to be collected for the *Family History,* it is necessary to have a clear understanding of the definition of the family. The family is defined in its broadest scope as two or more persons, sharing common goals and maintaining the following functions:

1. Bearing or adopting children and rearing them for independent living;

2. Providing shelter, food, clothing, health care, and safety measures;

3. Socializing family members by guiding the internalization of increasingly mature and acceptable patterns of behavior;

4. Allocating resources by apportioning goods, facilities, space, and other possessions;

5. Dividing labor by delineating to members of the family such responsibilities as providing income, managing the household, and caring for the family members; and

6. Providing motivation and meaning for family members by establishing ways of communication, rewarding members for achievement, meeting personal and family crises, and satisfying individual needs for acceptance.

Persons sharing these functions are usually joined by *ties of marriage, blood,* or *adoption.* However, there are increasing numbers of persons sharing these activities who are not married or consanguineous, for example, unmarried heterosexual or homosexual couples and persons living in a communal situation. The presence of a sexual tie is the distinguishing feature of a family versus friends, even though there may be no children involved. Therefore, the absence of a sexual relationship between friends who are living together precludes their being considered a family.

The data to be elicited about the family are its composition, the present health status of all members, familial illnesses, and relationships among family members. The specific data for each of these areas are outlined in Chart 8-1.

The importance of collecting data concerning the client's family centers around two major reasons. The first is that the family's health affects the individual as does his health affect the family. The effects could be physical— a contagious disease such as tuberculosis or venereal disease—or psychosocial problems related to stresses within the family. A child, for example, may be experiencing extreme anxiety due to the constant fighting of his parents and the impending threat of divorce. If such relationships are not assessed and needed intervention not provided, the child's anxiety might result in disruptive behavior or in a somatic illness. The second reason is that hereditary and constitutional factors are involved in the causation of certain conditions. It is through careful interviewing that the presence of familial illnesses can be detected and treated or that genetic counseling can be done to decrease the likelihood of the condition occurring. For instance, the mother of a child with diabetes mellitus has a lesion on her foot that is not healing. Although all the

CHART 8-1. Family History

Composition of family
    Relationship to client
    Age
    Sex

Health status of family members
    General description
    Present illnesses or injuries
    Other major stressors

Familial illnesses

Relationships among family members
    Roles
    Interactions

---

family members were assessed for diabetes at the time the child was diagnosed, the mother should be reassessed for the possibility of adult onset diabetes, since an early sign of this condition is delayed healing.

Composition

The specific members to be included in the *Family History* are:

1. Members of the nuclear or immediate family—parents, siblings, spouse, and children;
2. Members of the extended family—grandparents, grandchildren, aunts, uncles, and cousins; and
3. Significant others—heterosexual or homosexual partners and members of a commune.

The members of the nuclear family are considered in all aspects of the *Family History,* whether living in the same or in separate households. A son who is boarding at college is still considered in the father's *Family History.* Extended family members living in the same household are named specifically and are assessed in all aspects of the *Family History.* A mother-in-law, for example, who is an extended family member, not linked hereditarily, is not mentioned under familial illnesses. However, consanguineous members living outside the household are named only when referring to familial illnesses. If there are significant others, they are assessed under composition, health status, and relationships. They are not assessed under familial illnesses unless there are members of the nuclear family within the commune.

As each member is identified, his *relationship to the client* is recorded: father, wife, son, sister; next, *age* and *sex* are recorded. Obviously, sex need not be stated if the relationship clarifies this. However, when presenting cousins, the record should include the sex: "Cousin, 24-year old male, has a history of seizures." It is preferable in recording the *Family History* to present the members in descending chronological order—from the oldest to the youngest members. Although members are lost through death or severance of family ties, it is necessary to collect information regarding the cause of death or separation. If the member has died, his age at death, as well as the date and cause of death, if known, are recorded. A description of major factors surrounding the severance of family ties should be provided. It may be necessary to explain to the client why such information is needed before he will feel comfortable in discussing the exact reasons for a divorce or family disagreement. He may just say, "My son is no longer a part of the family. I don't know anything about his health." The client's right to privacy must be respected if he chooses to withhold information.

Health Status of Family Members

The health status of each family member is presented with a *general description of his health, present illnesses or injuries,* and *other major stressors.* The general description includes any physical, psychological, or social limitations due to past or present conditions. A brief statement of the problem and its effect on the client should be recorded: "My father is paralyzed in both legs since his car accident last year. Now I have to support the family." In another situation, the client tells you that his daughter has tuberculosis. You want to know what treatment his daughter is receiving, and what treatment other family members are receiving.

Major stressors, in addition to illnesses or injuries, that should be recorded include the death of a family member or friend; divorce; the loss of a job; the purchase of a new home; or the birth of a child. The stressors, whether positive or negative, can have a great influence on the health of the family members.

Familial Illnesses

Since hereditary and constitutional factors are involved in the causation of certain conditions, it is necessary to elicit information about the most frequently occurring ones. Although many diseases have not been considered genetically transmissible, a hereditary linkage may be suspected if other family members had, or presently have, a condition similar to that of the client.

There are two main reasons for obtaining this information. One is that genetic counseling may be offered to provide information about the nature of the illness already manifested, the risk of recurrence, and what a recurrence could mean. For example, parents may be concerned that another child will be born with a cleft lip or palate. Since there are several genetic and environmental factors involved, the probability is quite low that a subsequent child will be affected. In contrast, parents concerned about the recurrence of cystic fibrosis must be told that each child born to them has a 25 percent chance of having the disease, since it is caused by a single defective gene from each parent.

The second reason for a history of specific conditions is to alert the health personnel to the possibility that the present illness may be a hereditary disease or that the person or family should be screened for certain conditions so that early treatment may be instituted to prevent serious damage. If, for example, one child in the family has sickle cell anemia, the other children should be tested for signs of the disease, so that treatment can be instituted immediately.

Although there are close to 2000 identified inherited disorders and there are many more that appear to be familial, the main ones about which you specifically inquire are: hypertension, heart disease, cancer, diabetes mellitus, obesity, arthritis, gout, allergies, mental illness, renal disease, alcoholism, blood disorders, epilepsy, migraine, and the presence of jaundice or anemia. Of these conditions, some are definitely hereditary, such as blood disorders (hemophilia and sickle cell anemia) and certain forms of renal and heart disease. Yet there are others—most types of heart and renal diseases—of which only one of multiple determinants is hereditary. Some of these have questionable hereditary tendencies, including hypertension, allergies, obesity, and cancer. It is not known to what degree heredity is involved in diabetes mellitus and migraine.

The client's positive or negative response to each question is recorded, so that anyone who reads the history will know that you have questioned the client specifically about each one. Your notation includes any consanguineous member of nuclear or extended family who has, or has had, the condition, i.e. grandparents, grandchildren, aunts, uncles, cousins, siblings.

Relationships Among Family Members

First to be considered in assessing the relationships are the *roles* of each family member. Data about relationships among family members are of assistance in providing care or in identifying the causes of stress which can affect the client's health. For instance, knowing who performs the nurturing roles in the family aids in identifying the family member who should be most directly involved in a dietary teaching plan. A reversal of roles—the sustainer who suddenly becomes dependent—may produce additional stressors and affect the health of the entire family. The key roles within the family are: sustainer, nurturer, authority figure, counselor, and dependent. The degree to which each family member is involved in these roles varies. A father may be sustainer, nurturer, authority figure, and counselor. A member living outside the household may independently provide for his own needs and serve only as a counselor in the family. These data vary depending upon whether the family comprises a married couple with children, an unmarried heterosexual or homosexual couple, a single person with a child, or a communal group.

As the role of each member within the organization is identified, the client is asked to indicate whether, in his opinion, the role is appropriate and the member fulfills the role. Some specific questions that you might ask to elicit this information are:

Who provides the income for the family?
Who manages the household?
Who cares for the children?
Who disciplines the children?
How do the children assist with these activities?

The client may respond that both he and his wife work and that activities are equally divided between them. The client may say that he has been unable to work since his illness and that the children have all gone to work including the two oldest children who have dropped out of college, for the present time, to help with the financial situation.

The next point of information is the *interactions* among the family members. Ask the client to describe his interactions with family members and the interactions among the other members, including communication patterns and the general atmosphere of interactions—acceptance, rivalry, sharing. Also, the length of time the family spends together and their activities when they are together, e.g. meals, sports, church, travel, and how each participates. Ask the client to describe visits with relatives; the political, sexual or religious values of the members; recent or planned changes in the family, such as buying a new home, going to college, or a divorce in the family. When appropriate, information should be obtained concerning the client's sexual activity and satisfaction in it. As the client is describing the interactions within the family, the following and similar questions can direct his attention to the key areas:

How much time does the family spend together?
What activities are shared by the family?
Are possessions shared freely?
Does the family hold the same religious and political views?

An answer, "We get along well. There are no problems," should be pursued. What does "getting along well' and "with no problems" mean? It may mean that each one goes his separate way, and there is no time spent together, which may or may not be totally satisfying for the family members. If the client indicates that the family does not agree on many issues, follow-up questions could be: How does the family react to differing opinions? How does the family resolve conflicts?

Record of a Family History

The following record of a *Family History* will assist you in assimilating and utilizing the preceding data:

Family History: Mr. Rinehardt's father died of a heart attack in 1970 at the age of 65; he had no history of other illnesses. His mother, age 70, has hypertension which is being treated with a low sodium diet and diuretics. He has one brother, age 42, who has no history of illnesses, injuries, or major stressors. Mr. Rinehardt's wife, age 33, is in her seventh month of pregnancy, without complications. He has two children, a daughter, age 9, and a son, age 7, who have had no illnesses, injuries, or major stressors.

There is no other evidence of heart disease or hypertension in the family. He is not aware of the presence of cancer, diabetes mellitus, obesity, arthritis, gout, allergies, mental illness, renal disease, alcoholism, blood disorders, epilepsy, or migraine, or the presence of jaundice or anemia.

Mr. Rinehardt says that his roles are mainly "bread winner" and "the boss." His wife manages the house and cares for the children. The children "help with the chores and my daughter has a newspaper route." He feels that these are appropriate roles and that each person is fulfilling his role.

Mr. Rinehardt states that the family follows leisure-time activities together—camping, sailing, fishing and swimming. He says that they often go to movies and sometimes to plays. The general atmosphere of the interactions is one of acceptance and sharing. They visit both his and her relatives at least once a month. Both he and his wife share the same political and religious orientation, and have a satisfying sexual relationship. They are all "excited about the new baby."

This recording illustrates the kinds of information needed for the *Family History* and how adequate data organization can enable each member of the health care team to have an accurate understanding of the health status of the client's family.

Summary

The *Family History* appraises the physical, psychological, and social status of the client's family. This information is highly relevant, since an entire family can be affected by the illness of one member and because hereditary factors are involved in the causation of certain conditions. The *Family History* includes the composition of the family, the health status of the members, familial illnesses, and relationships among the members. Those considered are the nuclear family, the extended family, and significant others.

CHAPTER 9

sociAl histoRy

The *Social History,* which deals with social adjustments, provides information that directly influences the client's health and health problems and can be divided into three major elements: (1) relationships which occur outside of the family, (2) occupation/school, (3) environment, including factors within and outside the household. The specific data to be identified are outlined in Chart 9-1.

Perhaps this is a good time to reemphasize the importance of rapport established during the interview. The client may not appreciate the relation between the data collected in the *Social History* and his health. The personal nature of the information may make him reluctant to share it with you, so you may find it necessary to explain the reasons underlying these questions.

Relationships

Relationships outside the family are not always readily discerned because not everyone is cognizant

CHART 9-1. Social History

Relationships

Occupation/School
    Type of position
    Length of current position
    Conditions of employment/school
        Exposure to irritating or toxic agents
        Unusual environmental conditions
        Contact with various domestic or wild animals
        Pressures
    Relationships with peers and business associates
    Job or school satisfaction
    Financial status
    Past employment/school
        Types
        Conditions
        Dates or frequency of changes

Environment
    Types of living conditions
    Physical facilities
    Type of community
    Number of persons in household

---

of or sensitive to the manner in which he relates to others. Too, it may be difficult to formulate questions that will get at the specfic data. If the client is of school age, you might ask him to describe his school day: what he does in school, how he spends his recess or lunch time, and what he does after school. Children between the ages of six and seven have the need to relate to children of their own age, and they must have a "best friend." If a client of this age tells you that he spends his recess and lunch time reading a book and spends his time after school watching television alone, you would need to investigate why. It may be that the child has lived in an adult world and is rewarded only for his behavior or interactions with adults. Also, it could be that the child is a "loner" who will not interact with other children because he may not know how to or because he sees himself as different and fears teasing from his peers. Then, too, there is the possibility that parents will not allow their child to play with others and, therefore, the child has learned to be his "own friend."

    In exploring relationships with adults or adolescents it might be necessary to begin with childhood, then go on to evaluate each aspect of growth and development that is relative to the formation of relationships. It is between the ages of six and nine that one learns to make compromises with, to compete against, and to cooperate with one's peers. The preadolescent years are a time for learning to share ideas, to care for, and to accept others as readily as one does oneself. Skills needed for effective interaction with others develop at a very early age and progress through adolescence to maturity. Because the socialization process may be influenced at any point in time, the person may have difficulty in establishing adult relationships, or may reach maturity to realize abruptly that he cannot cope with them. A case in point would be the person who has married at a very young age; as his children near adolescence, he finds himself competing with them for attention and unable to cope with family responsibilities. Or it may be that the person has learned to interact and establish relationships only within his nuclear family, remaining unable to form relationships outside the family. Hence, in interviewing an adult, you might ask: "What types of activities do you engage in with your friends?" "What do you consider a friendship to be?" "Do you entertain your friends at home?" Asking questions such as: "Do you get along with others," may simply elicit the response "Yes." But do you know what he really means by the statement that he "gets along with others"?

Significant, too, is any abrupt change in relationships. A client may state that he always had many friends; enjoyed participating in group activities; was sought after by his friends as a confidant; and enjoyed discussing issues. However, suddenly he finds that he is irritable; his friends are shying away; he would much prefer to spend his time alone; and "people are too much of a bother—and besides, if you get involved with people you only get hurt!" A response such as this warrants further questioning. Is the client ill? Are friends shying away due to a change in his behavior? Is he spending time alone because of a financial problem, feeling too embarrassed to state that he cannot afford to participate in their activities? Are "people too much of a bother" because he is afraid of being hurt? Has he had a very painful relationship with which he cannot cope, and is he afraid of another deep involvement? Is he making life difficult for others because he harbors an unidentified anger resulting from past experiences? Could it be that he was not allowed to express his ideas or feelings during his early years, hence does not feel safe in doing so as an adult? The normal spontaneity of childhood may have been regarded as undesirable behavior, setting the stage for later inhibition.

Collecting data revolving around relationships could be both difficult and complicated. There may be a reluctance to share information that is seen as threatening or as an invasion of privacy. Nevertheless it has great significance to health status. The client's needs in this regard will be indicated by the data: a sudden change in behavior may suggest a brain tumor or a psychotic episode; long-standing interpersonal difficulties may require specialized counseling to get at the cause of the problem.

Occupation/School

It used to be thought that working conditions that affected health were those related only to long hours spent in cold, damp, dark, inadequately ventilated surroundings. We now know that irrespective of financial status or specific occupation, exposure to irritating or toxic agents, abnormal environmental conditions, and contact with domestic or wild animals have deleterious effects. You need to know about hours of work, also, as these could affect his health, as well as his relationship with his family. Physicians are generally regarded as being financially secure and enjoying a prestigious position within society, while rarely are their exposure to contagious diseases and their long hours of work mentioned; nor is the radiologist's exposure to radiation, with its potential for anemia, malignant tumors, and suppression of the bone marrow, often considered. In the manufacture of fluorescent lamps, beryllium is used; clothing worn by workers may be contaminated by the beryllium, and, when in contact with family members, may be the cause of berylliosis in them. Extremes of environmental temperatures have deleterious effects, too. Exposure to very high temperatures can lead to heat cramps, exhaustion, or stroke. Extreme cold can cause frostbite. Contact with both wild and domestic animals can result in rabies or allergies. Parrot fever is a viral infection carried by birds to man, so is important to consider if the client happens to be a pet shop owner.

These few examples should serve to underscore the importance of Occupational Data in the Health History.

One must also inquire whether occupation necessitates foreign or domestic travel. A salesman whose work takes him to Africa may be exposed to malaria. Persons who travel in Mexico may experience gastrointestinal disorders leading to dehydration and serious illness. And so on.

Along with obtaining data specifically related to exposure to toxins, irritants, or extreme environmental conditions, you will need to elicit data concerning length of current employment, past types of employment, and both physical and mental pressures. The data should also reflect how the client relates to his business associates and whether or not he enjoys his work.

Types and dates of past employment have relevance: Has the client changed jobs within the last six months? The problems he is presently experiencing may be related to previous environmental conditions or exposure to toxins. Has he worked in a poorly ventilated dry cleaning establishment? His extensive dermatitis, liver enlargement, and jaundice may be due to prior exposure to the carbon tetrachloride found in the cleaning fluid.

Although length of employment in itself may not bear on the client's health, it could certainly be signficant when considered along with information about business relationships and job satisfaction. Is the client changing jobs every few weeks because he cannot get along with people, or because he cannot find employment he enjoys and can do well?

Might he be unable to decide what type of work will enable him to be most productive? Does he live in a dream world, in which "the grass is always greener on the other side"? Perhaps his goals are unattainable, yet he has difficulty accepting this fact. Vocational guidance or counseling may be needed to help him deal with reality factors. In contrast, one tends to think that the client who has spent most of his working years at the same job enjoys his work, is productive, and gets along well with his co-workers. Yet, this is not necessarily true. Perhaps he was raised to believe that he should take a job and stay with it, whether or not he enjoys it. He is, at all costs, the "loyal employee." It might be a situation in which his loyalty was rewarded and he has moved up the ladder from a job in which he was comfortable and productive to one that is creating stress and consequently diminishing his productivity. One who has enjoyed productive employment and excellent relationships with his employer and co-workers may now find that he is not maintaining good relationships and that his productivity is decreasing. Is an organic lesion, such as a brain tumor, the cause? Of course, there are those who have planned their careers, changing jobs systematically, never stepping back or moving laterally, but always focusing on upward mobility.

It is clear that both physical and mental pressures may play a part; in fact, at times it is difficult to draw the line between the physical and the mental. A laborer doing heavy work may end each day physically exhausted yet feeling "very good" about his accomplishments; if that same person had a nagging boss, who was constantly pushing him, he could feel both physically and mentally exhausted. One who is bored might feel exhausted. Or, one who feels a constant need to achieve may be in a state of anxiety with resulting mental and physical exhaustion. Tensions associated with any work situation may give rise to numerous psychosomatic complaints. It is not unusual for a person in a stressful work situation—whether due to anxiety, competition, boredom, or fear of loss of employment—to seek health care, even though his complaint is not based on a physical problem. The most common complaint is fatigue, and the client appears depressed. Stressful work situations are thought to be one cause of such illnesses as the common cold. Sometimes you will hear the statement, "I didn't go to work today. I just needed a day to pull myself together—a mental health day." For the most part, pressures specifically related to occupation are not constant; often the person can plan accordingly. School teachers (and their students!) may feel tense at "term paper time"; accountants, as the April 15 income tax deadline looms; lawyers, when working on a particularly difficult case. Then, once the task is accomplished, the pressure decreases and the person resumes his normal pattern. He finds it difficult to cope only when the stress becomes great.

Financial pressure may revolve around family needs, rather than personal ones. In situations where families see themselves moving from one socioeconomic group to another, stress may be due to a desire for more income to "keep up with" the neighbors. If the financial situation affects status, this will in turn affect ego and self-esteem. External aspects of occupation do not always cause physical or mental stress.

Attending school is a child's main activity; it can give rise to much the same sort of stress as the adult work situation. The child is exposed to contagious diseases; competition among students may be keen, and personal relationships may be faltering. If the child is expected to produce beyond his capabilities, he may become tense. Mrs. Jones states:

> Brian started school at age two. It was just nursery school, he had to go, I had to work. He cried every day, in fact he still cries every day, but I make him go. I don't know why he cries; the other kids don't.

Brian may tell you:

> I don't like school.

Why? Is it because he never got over the fear of his mother leaving him? Is it because he does not do well in school? Is he afraid of the teacher? Do the children make fun of him? Is school work not seen as important within the family? Regardless of reason, the child may be experiencing anxieties that affect his health, and may need professional counseling to enable him to function and later meet the demands of a productive life.

As you begin to explore the school experience with a parent, you might be told:

> Cathy was an honor student until last year. Now she gets poor grades, doesn't want to go to school, and the teacher says she disturbs the whole class.

What does this mean? Why the sudden change? How does Cathy disturb the class? Has Cathy developed a physical problem that is interfering with her ability to function? Is Cathy upset because her parents are quarreling and talking about divorce? All of these need further investigation in order to help Cathy regain her previous level of functioning.

The adolescent may have other problems. Some may be typical "adolescent problems"; he may be more interested in extracurricular activities than academics; his parents may be pressuring him to follow one career whereas his interests lie elsewhere; he may be required to supplement the family income so cannot keep up with school work. And so on. If, in your opinion, his health is being impaired by school, then you must collect data that will enable you to identify the cause:

> At what age did you begin school?

Have you changed schools? Frequently?
Do you enjoy school?
How are you doing in school?
What kinds of activities do you participate in in school?
Do you have a part-time job? Does it affect your school work?
What are your career goals?
Do your parents support your career goals?

During the interview you may detect what could be considered an unhealthy attitude: a belief that everyone will be taken care of; no one needs to worry about working up to a potential; there is no need to worry about a job; there is no notion of responsibility to self or others. Counseling may be required.

Data about school may be recorded in this manner:

Sally started preschool at the age of four years. She cannot remember having problems adjusting to school; says she enjoys school and has always been an "honor student." Her parents are very supportive—help her with difficult assignments and always enjoy sharing her school interests, tales and activities. Sally works as a candy striper because "I want to and it gives me extra money to buy things I want." Presently, Sally is a senior in high school. She plans to attend college and study interior design. She says her parents "like the idea. They let me decorate my room last year."

You might conclude that school is having a positive effect on Sally's growth and development which affects her health; she does not appear to be under pressure, her parents are supportive, and they are not contributing to any anxieties that could impair her capacity to perform well.

Environment

Next to be dealt with is the Environmental History, which includes such factors as: type of habitat (house, apartment, commune); physical facilities (elevator, number of stairs, number of rooms, bathroom facilities); type of community (urban, rural); and number of persons in the household group.

A few examples will help you appreciate the influence of environment upon the client's health:

Mr. Allen is a twenty-five year old veteran of the Vietnamese war. As a result of injuries sustained during that war, he had a below-the-knee amputation of his right leg and a bowel resection which necessitated a colostomy. An infection developed in the right thigh which has become chronic and requires close supervision.

Mr. Allen may adjust well if he lives in a private, six room, ranch type home with two baths, in an urban community, and if the only other persons living in the household are his parents, with whom he has always enjoyed a supportive relationship of mutual concern, and if his friends visit him frequently.

However, if Mr. Allen lives in a five room walk-up apartment, on the fifth floor above the local general store in a rural community, and if he must share the apartment and its single bath with five family members, including his parents, a younger brother, and married sister and her husband, he may find adjustment difficult. Just the effort of walking up and down five flights of stairs can be very fatiguing, so he may choose to confine himself to the apartment, thereby cutting himself off from outside relationships. Sharing a bathroom with five other people is made even more difficult by his need for extra time for his colostomy care. The need for him to share a bedroom with his brother may cause him discomfort, since he must expose his physical disabilities to the brother. He needs privacy for his self-care. The number of people living in such crowded quarters may cause tension; the rural community may not provide the needed medical facilities. On the other hand, the family members may be so sensitive to his needs that they are *too* accommodating, and aggravate rather than lessen his discomfort.

This extreme example is not so unrealistic as it may seem. Health workers are often not aware that the client's environment is in any way different from their own. Without an accurate Environmental History, you might design an unrealistic plan for the client.

In Mr. Allen's case, it would be impractical to place him on a drug that necessitates a daily or weekly blood test if the community lacks adequate laboratory facilities; equally it would be impractical to prescribe total bed rest for a client who lives alone and has no nearby relatives, and whose closest neighbor lives 20 miles away. Conversely, the Environmental History may enable the health worker to plan for activities which the client would not otherwise have considered. The client may live in a large household where the social relationships provide much mutual concern and care. It might be of benefit to the health of an elderly client to have him cared for in his familiar environment, rather than to plan for nursing home care.

Recording the Social History

The *Social History* may be recorded in three parts; Relationships, Occupation/ School, and Environment. It should be concisely written and should contain data pertinent to the specific person. For example, if the client is an eight year old child, the *Social History* may read:

Relationships: Johnny has many friends with whom he plays baseball during his recess time and after school. He enjoys competitive games and says, "I don't always have to win." He is a member of the Cub Scouts and swims on the local community swim team. His friends come to his home for dinner and spend the night. He is also invited to their homes.

Occupation/School: Johnny is in the fourth grade. He has attended Public School 144 since first grade. He is an "average" student, but he "can do better." His mother says that both she and her husband try to reward him with money every time he does "very good work." It appears to her that when he wants money for something special, he will work. She feels he is smart and will pick up when school work has a "meaning." Johnny participates in school activities—class day, class play, parents' day, and sports events.

Environment: Johnny lives in a six room, single family, two-story home in an urban community with his parents and six-year old sister. He has his own bedroom and shares one of the two bathrooms with his sister.

The *Social History* for an adult may be more detailed:

Relationships: Ms. Taylor describes her relationships, until about six months ago, as being "very good." She has always had many friends, belonged to social and community groups, dated frequently, and had several experiences of "going steady." During her junior and senior years she was "pinned" and upon graduation, one year ago, she became engaged. Six months ago, she broke her engagement and moved to New York. Since that time, she has found it difficult to meet people, "get involved," and would rather spend her evenings reading. She says she is "not ready to be hurt again."

Occupation: Ms. Taylor has been employed for the past six months as a research biologist for a large pharmaceutical company. She works primarily with rats receiving radiation; the company keeps a close check on the amount of radiation to which employees are exposed. She described her work as being "fascinating"; the atmosphere is relaxed and casual; she enjoys her business associates. Her previous employment of six months was also as a research biologist testing drugs containing small amounts of arsenic. She left her previous employment to "get away," following her broken engagement. Her present job pays well and allows her to "live modestly but comfortably." She sees her present employment as a "step up" opportunity for upward mobility; and she will take advantage of the educational opportunities and become a "liberated career woman."

Environment: Ms. Taylor lives alone in a three room apartment on the tenth floor of an elevator building. The apartment consists of a small kitchen, large living-dining room, bath, and small bedroom, and she is conveniently located for shopping and public transportation. She feels the apartment adequately meets her needs, and her neighbors are young "business type" people who are friendly.

Ms. Taylor's *Social History* may seem rather lengthy but it contains pertinent data. What she has told you is that, until her broken engagement, she was popular and "related well" to people. Her ability to form relationships currently is associated with a recent experience that was painful and may be affecting her health. Her current and past employment is successful and is not influenced by her relationships, but may involve factors which could be deleterious to her health: working with rats; exposure to radiation; past exposure to arsenic. Her environment is conducive to "good" health and she is free of financial worries. Having this information will enable you to better evaluate Ms. Taylor's total health status.

Summary

The *Social History* is divided into three aspects—relationships, which occur outside of the family; occupation/school; and the effects of the environment which include factors within and outside the household. It includes data about the client's current social adjustments which provide information on the client's health. The recording of the *Social History* may be divided in relation to the three aspects.

CHAPTER 10

REViEW of SYSTEMS

The *Review of Systems* is the orderly assessment of the past and present status of the major anatomical areas of the body. This is the final component of the Health History, and serves as a verification that all relevant data have been obtained. It also groups together symptoms so that relationships among them can be readily identified. By asking the client specific questions about each system you may communicate the importance of each area to him, and assist him in recalling pertinent data. This may be just the stimulus the client needs to give you additional information explaining his *Reason for Contact* or, perhaps indicating a health need other than the one under evaluation.

The following episode illustrates this point. A client is admitted for a fractured hip which he sustained as a result of a fall. It is not until you are asking him if he has ever fainted that he says, "Yes, I have. In fact, I may even have fainted just before I fell. I don't know for certain." In questioning him further, you learn that he also has experienced infrequent cardiac palpitations. Since palpitations and syncope may result from complete heart block, his condition might be more serious than originally thought.

The *Review of Systems* must not be confused with the physical examination. The areas of assessment are similar, but the techniques used to obtain the data are different. The *Review of Systems* in the Health History is the informant's *verbal* response, via printed form, computer, or interview, to questions about each assessment area. The difference between the *Review of Systems* and the physical examination can be appreciated through the following example.

In reviewing material related to the neck, you ask the client if he has noticed any swelling or enlargement. He states that he has not noted any, but says, "The doctor told me that I have an enlarged thyroid." This would be recorded under the *Review of Systems.* Later, as you are doing the physical examination, you would palpate for any enlargement of the neck.

In the appraisal of each system, you should elicit a complete description of these areas:

1. Pain or discomfort, noting location, character, duration, and severity; and
2. Changes or disturbances in function.

The initial question for each system should be general, such as, "Have you had any difficulties with your eyes?" This permits the client to respond in what he considers to be the most salient manner to the assessment of his eyes. If the client's response does not provide information pertaining to the mentioned areas, you would then continue with specific questions similar to the following:

Have you had any pain or burning?
Have you ever had blurring of your vision?
Do you have any difficulty reading small print?

Both negative and positive responses are recorded to avoid later confusion about the presence or absence of certain symptoms. If there are positive responses, you would go on to ask additional questions about the occurrence of any associated symptoms. These questions are the same as those asked in the *Current Health Status:* date and time of onset; characteristics of the complaint; effects on activity patterns and body function; cause of the complaint, if known; treatment received, and the outcome. It is necessary to determine if symptoms are sporadic, frequent, or new. If the client had already given this information during data collection for the *Current Health Status,* do not repeat the questions. Furthermore, if the symptoms have been, or are, related to an illness or injury, the full description should appear in the appropriate component, either the *Past Health History* or *Current Health Status.* The notation in the *Review of Systems* would be a simple reference, such as:

Respiratory System:—Information about shortness of breath, hemoptysis and chest pain appears in the Current Health Status.

Body Systems

Before you begin the data collection, it is helpful to give the client an explanation by telling him that you will be asking a series of questions about various areas of his body in order to learn whether he has or ever had certain symptoms, conditions, examinations, or treatments that you have not yet discussed.

The systems to be assessed are:

General State of Health
Integumentary System
Head
Eyes
Ears
Nose and Sinuses
Mouth and Throat
Neck
Breast
Respiratory System
Cardiovascular System
Gastrointestinal System
Genitourinary System
Musculoskeletal System
Neurological System
Hematopoietic System
Endocrine System
Allergic and Immunological System

It is easier to remember the anatomical areas if one thinks of proceeding from "head to toe."

The first area of assessment in the *Review of Systems* is the client's General State of Health. This is a statement about *recent changes* in *weight* or *height* and *general well-being.* The specific symptoms about which you inquire are *weakness, fatigue, malaise, fever,* and *chills,* as these are manifestations of many disorders.

The Integumentary System, which includes the *skin, hair,* and *nails,* is the next area of assessment. The client is questioned specifically about *skin texture, excessive dryness* or *perspiration, alteration of temperature, pain, unusual pigmentation, rashes, pruritus, lesions,* and *growths.* When you ask the client about lesions, it is best to give some examples, such as blisters, wounds, ulcers, crusts, scales, so that he understands what is meant by the term. Inquire about *ab-*

normal growth, distribution, or *loss of hair* as well as the hair's *texture* and *condition.* The *shape, color,* and *condition* of the nails are elicited. These may be affected by changes in other parts of the body, as well as in the Integumentary System. For example, itching may be due to a drug reaction, biliary obstruction with jaundice, nephritis, or gout, to name a few.

An outline for assessment of the Integumentary System is:

Skin	*Hair*
1. Change in texture	1. Texture
2. Alteration in temperature	2. Condition
3. Excessive dryness or perspiration	3. Distribution
4. Unusual pigmentation	4. Abnormal growth or
5. Rashes	loss
6. Pruritus	*Nails*
7. Lesions	1. Shape
8. Growths	2. Color
9. Pain	3. Condition

The appraisal of the Head includes questions related to the presence of *pain* and *trauma.* A full description of headache, the most common symptom, should be given, noting character, severity, location, duration, associated symptoms, and measures that provide relief. Headache may be caused by disturbances in any body system. Headaches occurring infrequently are often related to fatigue, eyestrain, tension, acute febrile episodes, or dietary indiscretion. Chronic or recurrent headaches may be indicative of many conditions: intracranial tumor; infection; head injury; severe hypertension; disease of the eyes, nose, throat, and ears; migraine; allergies; uremia; alcoholism. The client's description might be similar to this one:

> *Head:* Mr. Hollander states that he does not remember ever being hit in the head, but did have "really bad" headaches for about four or five months at the end of last year. They started in the back of his head and spread all over it "like a pressure." He could not determine any cause. He was given Valium and told also to take aspirin. The headaches stopped after he changed jobs. (Information about stresses in his past employment is recorded in the Social History.) He was treated by Dr. M. Wayne, at Grundy Hospital, Grundy, Virginia.

Any other complaint, such as blurred vision, vertigo, tinnitus, or syncope, should be recorded in the appropriate place, e.g. Eyes, Ears, Neurological System.

Eyes are assessed for the presence of *itching, redness, edema, pain, diplopia, spots, blurring, lacrimation,* and *visual changes.* A notation is made of the type of visual changes, if known—hyperopia, myopia, astigmatism, strabismus, nystagmus.

If the *Reason for Contact* is for cataracts, the record for this part of the *Review of Systems* might read:

> *Eyes:* Mr. Endicott has experienced no itching, redness, edema, pain, or lacrimation. (A full description of symptoms due to cataracts appears in the Current Health Status.)

In reviewing the Ears, you inquire about the presence of *pain, discharge, hearing changes, vertigo,* and *tinnitus.* The following list presents some sample questions:

> Have you had any problems with your ears?
> Have you ever had earache or discharge from your ears?
> Did you ever note any ringing in your ears or dizziness?
> Have you been aware of any changes in your hearing?

Unless you are certain that the client will understand such words as tinnitus or vertigo, it is better to use "ringing in the ears" and "dizziness" when interviewing. If not, the client may just say "No," or "I don't know," rather than explain to you that he does not know the meaning of the words.

Symptoms referable to the Nose and the Sinuses include *pain, tenderness, discharges, obstruction* ("stuffiness"), *sneezing, changes in olfaction,* and *epistaxis.* Any discharge should be described as to its color, consistency, amount, and odor. If there is bleeding, the client is asked about precipitating factors, duration, amount, and presence of clots and drainage into his mouth.

A review of the Mouth and Throat includes a general question, followed by specifics:

> Did you ever have *pain, soreness,* or *lesions* of your tongue, gums, teeth, or throat?
> Do you have *difficulty chewing, tasting,* or *swallowing* food or liquids?
> Have you had any *hoarseness* or *changes* in your *voice?*

Positive responses are accompanied by a full description of the symptoms. For instance, if a client has dysphagia, you would want to know when he first noted the problem; his description of the complaint; how this has affected his diet; other activity patterns or body functions; his perception of its cause; what he has done to alleviate the problem, and whether this has been effective. The data to be collected are outlined in the following list:

Mouth and Throat

1. Pain	4. Altered taste
2. Soreness	5. Difficulty chewing
3. Lesions	6. Dysphagia

7. Bleeding	9. Hoarseness
8. Voice change	10. Condition of teeth

The next anatomical area to be assessed in the *Review of Systems* is the Neck. Inquiry should be made about *pain, swelling, enlargement,* and *limitations of movement.* The record might be similar to this:

> *Neck:* Mr. Peters has never noted any pain, swelling, enlargement, or limitation of movement.

Symptoms referable to the Breast include: *pain, tenderness, lumps, dimples, discharges,* and *changes in nipples.* A description of the breast *development* and *lactation,* if applicable, is obtained. Any findings of a breast self-examination are recorded.

The areas to be evaluated for the Respiratory System are:

1. Pain	4. Coughing
2. Dyspnea	5. Sputum
3. Wheezing	6. Hemoptysis

A positive response might lead to specific questions about illness, such as pneumonia, bronchitis, pleurisy, and tuberculosis, as well as the frequency and results of tuberculin skin tests and chest x-ray studies.

The following record is a complete assessment of the Respiratory System:

> *Respiratory System:* For the past three months Mr. Levis has had "a persistent, dry cough" which only occurs during the daytime. He has not sought any treatment since "it doesn't bother me." He reports no pain, dyspnea, wheezing, sputum, or hemoptysis.
>
> He says specifically that he does not smoke and has not had pneumonia, bronchitis, pleurisy, or exposure to tuberculosis. The tuberculin skin test and chest x-rays have been negative as is noted in the Past Health History.

In reviewing the Cardiovascular System, any *pain* should be fully assessed as to its location, character, severity, and duration. It is necessary to know if the pain is relieved by rest; this will assist you in differentiating angina pectoris from myocardial infarction. Similarly, any pain experienced in the extremities during walking (intermittent claudication) should be described. A full account of *dyspnea* should be reported—is the dyspnea noticed only upon exertion, such as when walking two flights of stairs or four blocks? Does he experience paroxysmal nocturnal dyspnea? Does he have orthopnea? Other symptoms about which you inquire are *palpitations, syncope,* and *edema.* The description of edema includes its location, degree, and relationship to any change in position.

The presence of any of these symptoms necessitates further investigation. The client is asked if he has ever been told that he had a heart murmur, hypertension, thrombophlebitis, or heart disease. A question that you might ask about examinations is: "Have you had any examination of the heart other than those you have already mentioned?" This serves a dual purpose: it provides the client with an opportunity to tell you about any additional tests such as cardiac catheterization and also lets him know that you have remembered his previous answers. If the client has received any drug therapy, especially medications such as nitroglycerin and digoxin, this fact is to be noted in the record.

The assessment of the Gastrointestinal System is extremely important in that many symptoms are indicative of problems not only within that system but in other body systems as well. For example, nausea and vomiting can be due to changes or disturbances in the gastrointestinal system itself or the inner ear, consequent to a head injury or an infection of the central nervous system. Similarly, anorexia and constipation, two other common symptoms, are often due to chronic depression, as well as to gastrointestinal disturbances.

One of the first symptoms to be assessed in this system is anorexia. You should note its severity and duration, and record any symptoms related to *food intake* or *intolerance*. A recent increase in appetite also can be diagnostic. This may occur in both diabetes mellitus and hyperthyroidism. It is not associated with a weight gain, rather, there is usually a weight loss in both of these conditions.

You continue your appraisal by asking the client about the presence of *nausea, vomiting, pyrosis, diarrhea, constipation, flatulence, jaundice,* and *change in bowel habits.* Any excretion—vomitus, drainage, stool—should be described as to its amount, character, color, and frequency. The presence of hematemesis and melena is to be noted.

The list that follows includes the major topics to be assessed in the Gastrointestinal System:

1. Pain
2. Pyrosis
3. Appetite changes
4. Food intolerance
5. Nausea
6. Emesis
7. Jaundice
8. Flatulence
9. Diarrhea
10. Constipation
11. Change in bowel habits

The data collected about the Genitourinary System encompass first a review of symptoms related to the Urinary Tract:

1. Dysuria
2. Burning
3. Urgency
4. Frequency
5. Hesitancy
6. Incontinence

7. Dribbling	10. Retention
8. Nocturia	11. Oliguria
9. Change in characteristics of urine	12. Polyuria

Since these terms may not be familiar to the client, it is preferable to ask questions that reflect a definition of the term. "Do you have difficulty in starting a stream?" is another way of asking, "Do you have hesitancy?" "Do you have to get up at night to urinate?" means "Do you have nocturia?" Changes in the characteristics of urine may be due to hematuria, pyuria, or sediment. Other changes in color may be caused by medications, diagnostic tests, or specific diseases. Incontinence of urine is described as to its frequency, occurrence during the day or night, and its relationship to activity.

The second area of assessment is the Genitalia. The symptoms apply to both males and females:

A. *General*

1. Pain	7. Sexual drive/activity
2. Burning	8. Sexual satisfaction
3. Lesions	9. Contraceptive methods
4. Edema	10. Impotence/frigidity
5. Discharges	11. Sterility
6. Secondary sex characteristics	

Any complaints of past or present pain, burning, lesions, or discharge are pursued further. Among other things, they may be related to venereal diseases, such as syphilis, gonorrhea, warts, or herpes genitalis.

Additional areas for investigation in the female involve:

B. *Menstrual/Menopausal*

1. Age at onset	7. Menorrhagia
2. Date of last period	8. Metrorrhagia
3. Amount of flow	9. Dysmenorrhea
4. Length of cycle	10. Cessation of menses
5. Duration	11. Hot flashes
6. Amenorrhea	

C. *Obstetrical*

1. Number of pregnancies	5. Complications of pregnancy
2. Deliveries; types	6. Miscarriages
3. Stillbirths	7. Abortions
4. Living children	

Questions about menstruation are important not only in assessing the integrity of the system, but also in identifying symptoms due to other conditions. Amenorrhea, for example, may be due to anorexia nervosa, pituitary tumor, hypothyroidism, or cirrhosis of the liver. Terms which might not be familiar to the client are not used except in recording, such as menorrhagia, metrorrhagia, and dysmenorrhea.

Symptoms referable to the Musculoskeletal System are: *pain, tenderness, cramps, swelling, weakness, deformities, decreased range of motion,* and *atrophy.* It is often difficult to determine whether certain symptoms—weakness is a good example—relate to primary muscle disease such as muscular dystrophy or to neurological conditions such as multiple sclerosis. However, upon identification of any symptom you must note the extremity and joint involved, whether it is unilateral or bilateral, and the effect on activity and locomotion, as well as any other relevant data.

The Neurological System is assessed by considering four statuses: general, mental, motor, and sensory. The first of these, the General Status, deals with symptoms related to the total system: *somnolence, vertigo, loss of consciousness, convulsions,* and *weakness.* These symptoms should be described as fully as possible. For example, the description for convulsions must include any earlier awareness of the approaching seizure; the parts of the body involved; the type and progress of movements; and the client's activity following the seizure. You should also inquire about the frequency of convulsions, the cause if known, and the treatment provided.

The Mental Status is considered next. Inquiry should be made about any *changes in disposition, insomnia, anxiety, amnesia, inability to meet responsibilities, difficulty in interactions, phobias, hallucinations,* and *depression.* A frequent complaint of clients is "nervousness"—a term that requires clarification because it can mean anxiety or fear to some, and tremors to others. It is during this part of the *Review of Systems* that the client might relate information about his relationships and interactions with family, friends, and business associates which he had not presented when questioned earlier. When asked about his ability to meet responsibilities, he may respond:

> I was doing quite well until last week. It wasn't until my boss said that I'd better shape up or he'd fire me, that I realized something was wrong. I know I can't work as fast now that I'm older as I used to, but I still get the work done. My wife blames everything on my drinking. I've been hitting the bottle more and more, but I really don't drink that much.

In this example, the client has indicated areas—occupation, family interactions, and drinking—that need to be investigated more completely. The focus on responsibility may have triggered the client's reactions, or perhaps he has become more comfortable with the interviewer. Regardless of the reason, since he is now divulging these data they should be pursued and should be recorded under the appropriate component.

The Motor Status is assessed for the presence of *difficulty in gait* or *coordination, tremors, paresis,* and *paralysis.* Questions you might ask are:

Have you had any trouble walking?
Do you ever feel clumsy or unsteady?
Do you frequently fall or bump into objects?
Did you ever have, or do you have, quivering or trembling in any part of your body?
Have you ever had a partial or complete loss of function in any extremity?

In appraising the Sensory Status, you inquire about *pain* and *paresthesia.* The client should describe any numbness, tingling, burning, or decreased sensation as specifically as he can. This helps to pinpoint the affected area of the Neurological System.

A sample record for the four statuses follows:

Neurological System:
General Status: Mr. Silverstein has had no vertigo, syncope, loss of consciousness, convulsions, or weakness.
Mental Status: He has noted no changes in his disposition, difficulties in interactions, amnesia, phobias, hallucinations, or depression. He does report "difficulty getting to sleep at night" and relates this to his job. There are no associated symptoms.
Motor Status: Mr. Silverstein relates no difficulty in gait or coordination, tremors, paresis, or paralysis.
Sensory Status: He has experienced no pain or paresthesia.

The Hematopoietic System is assessed by questioning the client about *bleeding tendencies, easy bruisability, lymph node enlargement,* and *exposure to toxic agents.* Some chemicals which can be toxic to the bone marrow are: benzene, dinitrophenol, trinitrotoluene, gold, arsenic, quinacrine, chloramphenicol, sulfonamides, and insecticides. The client is asked if he has ever had *anemia;* note the type, therapy, and response to treatment. Also record the client's *blood type,* if known.

The investigation of the Endocrine System considers all the endocrine glands, except the testes and ovaries, that have been included in the Genitourinary System. The glands manufacture hormones that control growth, metabolism, electrolyte and fluid balance, ability to cope with stress, and sexual development and function. Symptoms may result from either hyposecretion or hypersecretion of hormones. Many symptoms referable to this system have been presented throughout the *Review of Systems.* The main ones about which you would ask are:

1. Changes in:
   a. Skin
      (1) Texture
      (2) Pigmentation
      (3) Dryness or perspiration
   b. Hair distribution
   c. Weight and height
   d. Disposition
   e. Growth
   f. Sensitivity to temperature
2. Increased:
   a. Thirst (polydipsia)
   b. Appetite (polyphagia)
   c. Urine output (polyuria)
3. Anorexia
4. Weakness
5. Palpitations
6. Atrophy
7. Drowsiness
8. Goiter

If these have been recorded earlier, they need not be restated here.

The review of the Allergic and Immunological System considers: *pruritus, migraine, dermatitis, urticaria, angioedema, sneezing, vasomotor rhinitis,* and *conjunctivitis.* Any sensitivity to allergens should be noted along with type of reaction and time of year when it occurs. A notation in the client's record may be similar to this one:

> *Allergic and Immunological System:* Jimmy Barrett has had no pruritus, migraine, dermatitis, urticaria, angioedema, or conjunctivitis. He says, "I sneeze real bad and my nose runs whenever I mow the grass during the summer." He says that he has had no treatment for the allergy and has no other allergies. (A record of skin tests and immunizations appears in the Past Health History.)

Summary

The *Review of Systems,* the final component of the Health History, is the orderly assessment of the past and present statuses of the major anatomical parts of the body. The systems to be reviewed are:

General State of Health	Respiratory System
Integumentary System	Cardiovascular System
Head	Gastrointestinal System
Eyes	Genitourinary System
Ears	Musculoskeletal System
Nose and Sinuses	Neurological System
Mouth and Throat	Hematopoietic System
Neck	Endocrine System
Breast	Allergic and Immunologic System

In the assessment of each system you should elicit a complete description of these areas:

      1. Pain or discomfort, noting location, character, duration, and severity; and

      2. Changes or disturbances in function.

The initial questions related to each system should be general and should be followed by more specific ones. The main data that should be elicited are presented with each system. Both negative and positive responses are recorded. Positive responses are accompanied by a full description of the symptoms: date and time of onset; characteristics of the complaint; associated symptoms; effects on activity patterns and body functions; cause of the complaint, if known; examination, including the date, time, place, examiner, and significant findings; and treatments, for instance, medications, prostheses, and surgical procedures.

The *Review of Systems* serves as a final check that all relevant data have been collected; it groups together symptoms for easier identification of relationships among them; and it provides an opportunity for the client to present additional data. When all information has been collected, the Health History is complete.

PART III

APPENdices

appendix a

outline guide
for the collection of
a health history

Date

I   REASON FOR CONTACT

Reason for encounter with health personnel and facility.

II   BIOGRAPHICAL DATA

    A.   Full name
    B.   Residence
    C.   Telephone Number
    D.   Age
    E.   Date of Birth
    F.   Place of Birth
    G.   Sex
    H.   Ethnic Group
    I.   Religion
    J   Primary Spoken Language
    K.   Marital Status

109

- L. Education
- M. Occupation
- N. Health Insurance
- O. Social Security Number
- P. First Names of Parents; Mother's Maiden Name

III   CURRENT HEALTH STATUS

- A. *Details of Specific Complaint*
- B. *Daily Habits and/or Activity Patterns*

1. Diet
2. Elimination
3. Personal Hygiene
4. Use of Tobacco and Drugs
5. Recreation and Exercise/Play
6. Sleep

IV   PAST HEALTH HISTORY

- A. *Developmental Data*
- B. *Promotive and Preventive Practices*

1. Examinations
2. Counseling
3. Immunizations

- C. *Restorative Interventions*

1. Past Illnesses, Injuries, and Surgery
2. Infectious Diseases

- D. *Allergies*
- E. *Foreign Travel*

V   FAMILY HISTORY

- A. *Composition of Family*

1. Relationship to Client
2. Age
3. Sex

- B. *Health Status of Family Members*

1. General Description
2. Present Illnesses or Injuries
3. Other Major Stressors

- C. *Familial Illnesses*
- D. *Relationships Among Family Members*

1. Roles
2. Interactions

VI SOCIAL HISTORY

 A. *Relationships*
 B. *Occupation/School*

 1. Type of Position
 2. Length of Current Position
 3. Conditions of Employment/School
  (a) Exposure to irritating or toxic agents
  (b) Unusual environmental conditions
  (c) Contact with various domestic or wild animals
  (d) Pressures
 4. Relationships with Peers and Business Associates
 5. Job or School Satisfaction
 6. Financial Status
 7. Past Employment/School
  (a) Types
  (b) Conditions
  (c) Dates or frequency of changes

 C. *Environment*

 1. Types of Living Conditions
 2. Physical Facilities
 3. Type of Community
 4. Number of Persons in Household

VII REVIEW OF SYSTEMS

 A. *General State of Health*

 1. Recent Change in Weight and Height
 2. Weakness
 3. Fatigue
 4. Malaise
 5. Fever
 6. Chills

 B. *Integumentary System*

 1. Skin
  (a) Texture   (e) Pruritus
  (b) Excessive dryness or perspiration (f) Lesions
  (c) Alteration in temperature (g) Growths
  (d) Unusual pigmentation

2. Hair
   (a) Texture
   (b) Condition
   (c) Distribution
   (d) Abnormal growth or loss

3. Nails
   (a) Shape
   (b) Color
   (c) Condition

C. *Head*

1. Pain
2. Trauma

D. *Eyes*

1. Itching
2. Redness
3. Edema
4. Pain
5. Diplopia
6. Blurring
7. Spots
8. Lacrimation
9. Visual Changes

E. *Ears*

1. Pain
2. Discharges
3. Hearing Changes
4. Vertigo
5. Tinnitus

F. *Nose and Sinuses*

1. Pain
2. Tenderness
3. Discharges
4. Obstruction
5. Sneezing
6. Olfactory Changes
7. Epistaxis

G. *Mouth and Throat*

1. Pain
2. Soreness
3. Lesions
4. Altered Taste
5. Difficulty in Chewing
6. Dysphagia
7. Bleeding
8. Voice Changes
9. Hoarseness
10. Condition of Teeth

H. *Neck*

1. Pain
2. Swelling
3. Enlargement
4. Limitation of Movement

I. *Breast*

1. Pain
2. Tenderness
3. Lumps
4. Dimples

5. Discharges
6. Changes in Nipples

7. Development
8. Lactation

J. *Respiratory System*

1. Pain
2. Dyspnea
3. Wheezing

4. Coughing
5. Sputum
6. Hemoptysis

K. *Cardiovascular System*

1. Pain
2. Dyspnea
3. Palpitations

4. Syncope
5. Edema

L. *Gastrointestinal System*

1. Pain
2. Pyrosis
3. Appetite Changes
4. Food Intolerance
5. Nausea
6. Emesis

7. Jaundice
8. Flatulence
9. Diarrhea
10. Constipation
11. Change in Bowel Habits

M. *Genitourinary System*

1. Urinary Tract
   (a) Dysuria
   (b) Burning
   (c) Urgency
   (d) Frequency
   (e) Hesitancy
   (f) Incontinence

   (g) Dribbling
   (h) Nocturia
   (i) Change in character- istics of urine
   (j) Retention
   (k) Oliguria
   (l) Polyuria

2. Genitalia
   (a) Pain
   (b) Burning
   (c) Lesions
   (d) Edema
   (e) Discharges
   (f) Secondary sex characteristics

   (g) Sexual drive/activity/ satisfaction
   (h) Contraceptive methods
   (i) Impotence/frigidity
   (j) Sterility

3. Menstrual/Menopausal
   (a) Age at onset
   (b) Date of last period
   (c) Amount of flow
   (d) Length of cycle
   (e) Duration
   (f) Amenorrhea

   (g) Menorrhagia
   (h) Metrorrhagia
   (i) Dysmenorrhea
   (j) Cessation of menses
   (k) Hot flashes

4. Obstetrical
    (a) Number of pregnancies
    (b) Deliveries; types
    (c) Stillbirths
    (d) Living children
    (e) Complications of pregnancy
    (f) Miscarriages
    (g) Abortions

N. Musculoskeletal System

1. Pain
2. Tenderness
3. Cramps
4. Swelling
5. Weakness
6. Deformities
7. Decreased Range of Motion
8. Atrophy

O. Neurological System

1. General Status
    (a) Somnolence
    (b) Vertigo
    (c) Loss of consciousness
    (d) Convulsions
    (e) Weakness
2. Mental Status
    (a) Changes in disposition
    (b) Insomnia
    (c) Anxiety
    (d) Amnesia
    (e) Inability to meet responsibilities
    (f) Difficulty in interactions
    (g) Phobias
    (h) Hallucinations
    (i) Depression
3. Motor Status
    (a) Altered gait
    (b) Difficulty in coordination
    (c) Tremors
    (d) Paresis
    (e) Paralysis
4. Sensory Status
    (a) Pain
    (b) Paresthesia

P. Hematopoietic System

1. Bleeding Tendencies
2. Easy Bruisability
3. Lymph Node Enlargement
4. Exposure to Toxic Agents
5. Anemia
6. Blood Type

Q. Endocrine System

1. Change in Skin Texture
2. Excessive Dryness or Perspiration
3. Unusual Pigmentation
4. Abnormal Hair Distribution
5. Change in Weight and Height
6. Sensitivity to Temperature Variations
7. Change in Disposition

8. Abnormal Growth
9. Polydipsia
10. Polyphagia
11. Polyuria
12. Anorexia

13. Weakness
14. Drowsiness
15. Palpitations
16. Atrophy
17. Goiter

R. Allergic and Immunological System

1. Pruritus
2. Migraine
3. Dermatitis
4. Urticaria

5. Sneezing
6. Angioedema
7. Vasomotor Rhinitis
8. Conjunctivitis

appendix b-1

A complete HEALTH history

DATE: September 20, 1975

REASON FOR CONTACT

"I've had a dull pain under my diaphragm, nausea, and hot and cold chills for the last five hours."

BIOGRAPHICAL DATA

Theresa Anne Borden lives at 214 Highland Drive, Oak Hills, Wisconsin, 54922. Her phone number is 414-734-1234. She is a thirty-year old, single English-speaking woman of Irish-German descent and was born in Boston, Massachusetts on June 25, 1945. She is Roman Catholic, has a Master's degree and teaches college Mathematics; English is her primary language. She has Blue Cross-Blue Shield Health Insurance and her Social Security number is 033-30-4774. Her father's name is Charles Michael and her mother is Dorothea Anna, nee Ringer.

CURRENT HEALTH STATUS

Complaint: She reports a "dull, gnawing pain" under her diaphragm, which started about 8:30 a.m. It is "uncomfortable, but bearable"; She was able to work for about two hours and then began to have hot and cold chills. The symptoms were not relieved by two aspirin nor by rest. She states: "I really feel lousy."

Diet: Ms. Borden states that she has a "good" appetite, although today she has not felt like eating anything since breakfast, because of her nausea. She is 5 feet 2 inches tall, and weighs 112 pounds which she says is "right for me." Her maximum weight was 128 pounds at age 20 and minimum weight was 105 pounds at age twenty-six, during graduate school. Her daily food intake consists of juice, two cups of coffee and cereal for breakfast; a meat or fish sandwich, fruit and decaffeinated coffee for lunch; meat or fish, two vegetables, ice cream or fruit, and milk for dinner; and occasional snacks of fruit, ice cream or potato chips in the evening. She drinks approximately three cups of regular or decaffeinated coffee and four glasses of water between meals daily. She eats "everything," feels most hungry around dinner and in the evening, has no restrictions on her diet and has never been on a diet. She prepares her own meals and frequently—three or four times a week—eats at home or "out" with friends.

Elimination: She has a bowel movement daily after breakfast; it is a brown, soft and formed stool with no unusual odor. Occasionally she skips a day but does not see that as a problem. Ms. Borden voids about five times a day; it is clear, light yellow, no odor.

Personal Hygiene: She takes a bath or shower each evening, washes her hair once a week, brushes her teeth twice a day and manicures her nails twice a week.

Tobacco and Drugs: She has smoked a pack of cigarettes a day for the last eight years. She does not use sedatives, barbiturates, narcotics, amphetamines, or laxatives. She takes two aspirin for headaches but no other medication. She drinks about two scotches or martinis a week.

Recreation and Exercise: She relates that she has many interests: reading, attending plays, knitting, swimming, watching basketball and football, playing tennis and basketball weekly "in season," traveling and "seeing new places," which she does yearly on a four week vacation and about one weekend a month. She has a "large slide collection of travels, family and friends."

Sleep Patterns: She sleeps about seven hours a night without interruption, falls asleep without difficulty, and feels rested on awakening. When she is really busy, she "gets by on four or five hours" but then sleeps late on the weekend or takes a nap before going out in the evening.

PAST HEALTH HISTORY

Developmental Data: Ms. Borden relates no developmental problems.

Promotive and Preventive Practices: She has a yearly physical examination, including chest x-ray, "Pap" smear, blood work and urinalysis. The last one was on June 5, 1975 by Dr. R. Peters at Middle State Medical Center, Oak Hills, Wisconsin. All findings were "negative." Ms. Borden has semiannual dental exams with Dr. T. Carey, also at the Medical Center; her last exam on July 10, 1975 revealed no cavities. Her eyes are examined every two years by Dr. M. Smile, 10 Winter Street, Boston, Massachusetts. Her next appointment is over the Christmas holidays. She performs a monthly breast self-examination after her periods.

Her last immunizations were: Diphtheria, pertussis, tetanus in January 1960; Salk vaccine in April, 1965 and Sabin vaccine in August, October and December, 1968; cholera and tetanus in June, 1969; and smallpox, typhoid and a tuberculin skin test (with positive results) in July, 1973. She has received no immunizations against measles or mumps.

Restorative Intervention: Her infectious disease history includes "regular" measles and mumps in 1949 and chicken pox and pertussis in 1950. In 1951 she had bronchial pneumonia which was treated by "hospitalization for about two weeks and penicillin" at Children's Hospital in Boston. She remembers no other specifics. She denies having had rheumatic fever, malaria, scarlet fever, diphtheria, poliomyelitis, and tuberculosis.

In 1949 she had a tonsillectomy and adenoidectomy, also at Children's Hospital; she thinks that she was hospitalized for two days but does not remember anything else.

In May, 1972, she was hospitalized for two days for a dilatation and curettage and the removal of polyps under general anesthesia at Chase Hospital in Boston. Her surgeon was Dr. J. Baker. She received "routine" vitamin K, one day postsurgery and returned to work after one week, although she felt tired for the next month.

She has no known allergies. She received penicillin with no adverse effect and has never had a blood transfusion.

Foreign travel: Ms. Borden enjoys traveling and visited Utah, Arizona and Nevada this past summer.

FAMILY HISTORY

Her maternal grandfather died of cancer of the liver in 1945 when he was 65 years old; her maternal grandmother died in 1959 at the age of 80; after "several heart attacks." Her father died in a car accident in 1949 at the age of 38; he had no known illnesses. Her mother, age 60, had a "heart attack" in 1965 but has had no illnesses or injuries since. She was "very happy" to become a grandmother two months ago. Her sister, age 32, has no history of illnesses or injuries. She gave birth to her first child, a son, two months ago; that was a "happy" occasion for all the family.

There is no other evidence of heart disease or cancer in the family. She knows of no family members having hypertension, diabetes mellitus, obesity, arthritis, gout, allergies, mental illness, renal disease, alcoholism, blood disorders, epilepsy, migraine, jaundice or anemia.

Ms. Borden states that she is independent but "close" to her family despite the geographical distance. She talks with her family every other week and they visit four times a year. They share the same religious views but occasionally differ on political issues; each feels free to discuss his positions and adhere to them.

SOCIAL HISTORY

Relationships: Ms. Borden states that she gets along "well with others." She has four "very close" friends, as well as many acquaintances. She dates but does not "feel any pressure to marry." She is active in local elections.

Occupation: She has been teaching at Middle State College for two years. She enjoys her job, colleagues and students; is a member of several committees and relates that her work is not stressful. She also is finishing her doctoral dissertation and hopes to receive her degree in the spring. She is not exposed to any toxic agents, unusual conditions, or wild animals.

She states that her salary is "good"—she lives "comfortably," and has enough money to travel for a month each year and still add to her savings account.

Formerly she taught for two years in a community college near Boston, Massachusetts. She describes the situation as "rough," in terms of student-faculty ratio and with little involvement in decision-making.

Environment: She lives alone in a "comfortable" four room apartment, on the second floor of a two family house, in a suburban community. The apartment consists of a kitchen, bedroom, den/guest room, large living room, bathroom, and porch. Stores and church are within a five minute drive. Her neighbors are described as young to middle aged singles and families who are very friendly and helpful.

REVIEW OF SYSTEMS

General State of Health: Ms. Borden has had no recent changes in either weight or height and usually feels "good." Today she feels weak, "drained and lousy," has hot and cold chills, as indicated in Current Health Status. She seldom has fevers, except with a "bad cold" and does not know if she has one today.

Integumentary System: She describes her skin as soft, elastic, her feet are occasionally dry in the winter but "lotion softens them." She usually perspires more in warm weather only, but today feels "clammy." She denies any pain, unusual alterations of temperature or pigmentation, rashes, pruritus, lesions or growths. She relates no abnormal hair growth, distribution or loss or changes in nails.

Head: She says that she has a headache about once a month which she relates to being overtired and which is relieved by two aspirin. She has had no head injury.

Eyes: She denies itching, redness, edema, diplopia, spots, blurring and lacrimation. She wears glasses for reading.

Ears: She relates no pain, discharges, hearing changes, vertigo or tinnitus.

Nose and Sinuses: She claims no pain, tenderness, discharges, sneezing, obstruction, changes in smelling or epistaxis.

Mouth and Throat: She denies pain, soreness, lesions, altered taste, difficulty in chewing or swallowing; bleeding, voice changes and hoarseness ("unless I've been lecturing for a few hours"). She has no dentures or caries.

Neck: She has never noted pain, swelling, enlargement or limited movement.

Breast: She denies pain, tenderness, lumps, dimples, discharges and changes in nipples.

Respiratory System: She states that she has no pain, dyspnea, wheezing, coughing, sputum or hemoptysis.

Cardiovascular System: She relates no pain, dyspnea, palpitations, syncope or edema.

Gastrointestinal System: She denies pyrosis, change in appetite, food intolerance, emesis, jaundice, flatulence, diarrhea, constipation and change in bowel habits. A description of pain and nausea is included in the Current Health History.

Genitourinary System

Urinary tract: She states that she has no dysuria, burning, urgency, frequency, hesitancy, incontinence, dribbling, change in color, nocturia, retention, or oliguria.

Genitalia: She denies pain, burning, lesions, edema and abnormal discharges. Her breasts enlarged and pubic hair appeared when she was "twelve or thirteen years old." She says that she does not masturbate and has not had sexual intercourse—"sex belongs with marriage."

Menstrual/menopausal: She relates that menstruation began at age eleven. Her last period was August 20, 1975. Her cycle is 28 days, lasting for seven days, with a heavy flow for the first four days. She had one episode of metrorrhagia due to polyps in 1972. (Details are noted in Past Health History.)

She denies amenorrhea, menorrhagia, dysmenorrhea, hot flashes and onset of menopause.

Obstetrical: She has had no pregnancies.

Musculoskeletal System: She denies pain, tenderness, cramps, swelling, weakness, deformities, decreased range of motion and atrophy.

Neurological System:

General Status: She has no vertigo, somnolence, loss of consciousness convulsions or weakness.

Mental status: She claims no changes in disposition, insomnia, anxiety, amnesia, inability to meet responsibilities, difficulty in interactions, phobias, hallucinations or depression.

Motor status: She denies difficulty in gait or coordination, tremors, paresis and paralysis.

Sensory status: She relates no pain or paresthesia.

Hematopoietic System: She denies anemia, bleeding, tenderness, easy bruisability, lymph node enlargement and exposure to toxic agents. Blood type unknown.

Endocrine System: She claims no goiter, polydipsia, polyuria, or polyphagia.

Allergic and Immunologic System: She has no pruritus, migraine, dermatitis, urticaria, angioedema, sneezing, vasomotor rhinitis, conjunctivitis, or sensitivity to allergens.

Jean Nichols, R.N.

appendix b-2

A COMPLETE HEALTH HISTORY

DATE: August 29, 1975

REASON FOR CONTACT:

Mother states, "John needs a school physical."

BIOGRAPHICAL DATA

John Paul Andrews lives at 10 Main Street, Riverdale, New York, 10001. His telephone number is 212-123-4567. He is a seven-year old, English speaking male student born in Columbus, Ohio, September 10, 1968 and is of English-Scottish background. He attends the Presbyterian Church. His parents, Paul and Mary Smith Andrews, have Blue Cross Insurance (family plan).

CURRENT HEALTH STATUS

John has come to the clinic for his yearly school physical. His mother reports that he has not been sick.

Diet: Mrs. Andrews states that John weighs about 51 pounds and is 48 inches tall; he has never been under- or overweight. His diet consists of eggs or cereal, milk and juice for breakfast; cheese, peanut-butter or a meat sandwich or soup, milk and gelatin for lunch; meat, vegetables, potatoes or rice, milk and fruit for dinner. He "isn't a big sweets eater"; prefers to snack on potato chips; rarely drinks water, but does drink about three glasses of juice during the day. He likes all foods, has no allergies or food intolerence. She has never had a problem with John's eating.

Elimination: John has a bowel movement every day which he says is "brown and normal." He does not know how many times he voids daily, "maybe five times" and his urine is "yellow and smells right."

Personal Hygiene: John takes a bath every evening; brushes his teeth after breakfast and before going to bed. His mother washes his hair once a week and "scrubs" his nails daily.

Tobacco and Drugs: He takes no drugs.

Recreation and Exercise: John has "lots of hobbies—collects rocks, baseball cards and miniature cars." He plays baseball or bike rides with his friends every-day; has a pet rabbit which he cares for and belongs to the Cub Scouts. He also takes horseback riding lessons.

Sleep Patterns: John goes to bed at 8 p.m., has no trouble falling asleep, is occasionally awakened by a "bad dream." He awakens at 7 a.m.; he says he feels "good" when he gets up, is never tired and does not nap.

PAST HEALTH HISTORY

Developmental Data: John's mother states that he has had no developmental difficulties. He readily adjusts to new situations—"even our move a year ago."

Promotive and Preventive Practices: John had a school physical, dental and ophthalmic examination on July 31, 1974, at the Group Clinic, 20 Allen Street, Columbus, Ohio. He had no counseling services. His immunizations, all done at the Group Clinic are:

1. Diphtheria, tetanus, pertussis and polio vaccine at two, four, and six months of age and when two and six years old;
2. Rubeola and tuberculin skin test at one year of age; and
3. Mumps and rubella at six years.

Restorative Intervention: He had "three day measles" in 1972 and chicken pox in 1973, without complications. His mother states that he has had no injuries, surgery, rheumatic fever, malaria, scarlet fever, diphtheria, rubeola, mumps, poliomyelitis, tuberculosis or pertussis.

Allergies: He had had no known allergies. He has not had penicillin or a blood transfusion.

Foreign Travel: He vacationed with his family in England, France and Germany during this past June and July.

FAMILY HISTORY

His paternal grandfather died, at age sixty-four, of a "heart attack" in 1973; his paternal grandmother, age sixty-seven, had a radical mastectomy in 1975. She has no other illnesses, injuries, or surgery. John's maternal grandfather, age sixty-eight, has hypertension which is being treated with diet and diuretics. His maternal grandmother has angina pectoris for which she takes nitroglycerin. John's father, age thirty, his mother, age twenty-eight, and a sister, age six, have no illnesses, injuries, or other major stresses.

There is no evidence in the family of diabetes mellitus, obesity, arthritis, gout, allergies, mental illness, renal disease, alcoholism, blood disorders, epilepsy, migraine or the presence of jaundice or anemia.

Though John is young, he assists with household tasks. John states that he and his sister get along well except for "a few good fights." The mother states that "we are a close family" and do many activities together—meals, watching television, vacationing and church. They visit the father's family about twice a year since they live about 300 miles away. The mother's family live close by and are visited weekly.

SOCIAL HISTORY

Relationships: He has many friends with whom he plays during his recess time and after school. He enjoys games, but says "I don't have to always win." He is involved in group activities and presently is captain of the baseball team. His friends visit his home, sometimes spend the night, and he is invited to their homes.

Occupation/School: John is in the third grade at Drew School. He likes school and his mother says that he is an "excellent" student, has no problems and that she and her husband participate in school activities and help John with his homework.

Environment: John lives in a six room, one family, two story home in a suburban area, with his parents and six year old sister. He has his own bedroom and shares one of two baths. He says his friends like to come and play at his house because they always have a good time.

REVIEW OF SYSTEMS

General State of Health: During the last year, John has grown two inches and gained three pounds. He denies any weakness, fatigue, malaise, fever or chills.

Integumentary System

Skin: He has had no change in texture, pigmentation, temperature, or moisture of skin. He denies pruritus, lesions, rashes or growths.

Hair: No change in texture, condition, or distribution has been noted. There has been no abnormal growth or loss.

Nails: He relates that there has been no change in shape, color and condition.

Head: He denies ever having headaches or injuries.

Eyes: He claims no itching, redness, edema, pain, tearing, blurring, spots, diplopia, or visual changes.

Ears: John relates that he has had no earaches, discharge, vertigo, or tinnitus. He says, "I can hear anything."

Nose and Sinuses: He denies any pain, tenderness, obstruction, sneezing, or epistaxis. He states that his "nose only runs when I have a cold." He has no difficulty smelling.

Mouth and Throat: He does not get frequent sore throats—"just a little soreness about once a year." He denies any lesions, pain, change in taste, dysphagia, bleeding, difficulty chewing, hoarseness or voice changes. He says that he does not think he has any cavities, but "I did have one filled last year."

Neck: He has noted no pain, swelling, enlargement or limitation of movement.

Respiratory System: He denies pain, dyspnea, wheezing, coughing, sputum or hemoptysis.

Cardiovascular System: He claims no pain, dyspnea, palpitation, syncope or edema.

Gastrointestinal System: He has not noted any pain, pyrosis, nausea, emesis, jaundice, flatulence, diarrhea, constipation or change in bowel habits. His mother says, "He can eat anything."

Genitourinary System

Urinary Tract: He claims no burning, dysuria, urgency, frequency, incontinence, dribbling, change in characteristics of urine, hesitancy, retention, or oliguria. He says, "I always go at night if I drink too much juice before going to bed."

Genitalia: He relates no pain, burning, lesions, edema, or discharge. His mother states she is unaware of any masturbation.

Musculoskeletal System: He denies any pain, tenderness, cramps, swelling, weakness, deformities, decreased range of motion or atrophy.

Neurological System

General Status: He relates no somnolence, vertigo, loss of consciousness, convulsions or weakness.

Mental Status: His mother says that he has no changes in disposition, insomnia, anxiety, amnesia, inability to meet responsibilities, difficulty in interactions, hallucinations or depression. She states that he is afraid of heights and "won't even climb trees."

Motor Status: He has noted no difficulty in gait or coordination, tremors, paresis or paralysis.

Sensory Status: He relates no pain or paresthesia.

Hematopoietic System: He denies any bleeding tendencies, easy bruisability, lymph node enlargement, exposure to toxic agents, or anemia. Blood type unknown.

Endocrine System: He denies polydipsia, polyphagia and polyuria.

Allergic and Immunologic System: He claims no pruritus, migraine, dermatitis, urticaria, angioedema, sneezing, vasomotor rhinitis, conjunctivitis or sensitivity to allergens.

Mary Barone, R.N.

bibliogRAPhy

Barness, Lewis A. *Manual of Pediatric Physical Diagnosis.* 2nd ed. Chicago: Year Book Medical Publishers, Inc., 1971.

Bernstein, Louis and Dana, Richard H. *Interviewing and the Health Professions.* New York: Appleton-Century-Crofts, 1970.

Bonkowsky, Marilyn L. "Adapting the POMR to Community Child Health Care." *Nursing Outlook,* 20 (August, 1972), 515–518.

Brantl, Virginia M. and Brown, Marie Raymond. *Readings in Gerontology.* Saint Louis: The C.V. Mosby Company, 1973.

Carlson, Carolyn E. *Behavioral Concepts and Nursing Intervention.* Philadelphia: J.B. Lippincott Company, 1970.

Chinn, Peggy L. and Leitch, Cynthia J. *Child Health Maintenance, A Guide to Clinical Assessment.* Saint Louis: The C.V. Mosby Company, 1974.

DeAngelis, Catherine. *Basic Pediatrics for the Primary Health Care Provider.* Boston: Little, Brown and Company, 1975.

DeGowin, Elmer L. and DeGowin, Richard L. *Bedside Diagnostic Examination.* 2nd Edition. New York: MacMillan Publishing Co., Inc., 1971.

Diekelmann, Nancy and Galloway, Karen. "A Time of Change." *American Journal of Nursing,* 75 (June, 1975), 994–996.

Erikson, Erik H. *Childhood and Society.* New York: W.W. Norton & Company, Inc., 1964.

Fowkes, William C., Jr. and Hunn, Virginia K. *Clinical Assessment for the Nurse Practitioner.* Saint Louis: The C.V. Mosby Company, 1973.

French, Ruth M. *The Dynamics of Health Care.* 2nd ed. New York: McGraw-Hill Book Company, 1974.

Froehlich, Robert E. and Bishop, F. Marian. *Medical Interviewing: A Programmed Manual.* 2nd ed. Saint Louis: The C.V. Mosby Company, 1972.

Harvey, A. McGehee, Johns, Richard J., Owens, Albert H., and Ross, Richard S.

The Principles and Practice of Medicine. New York: Appleton-Century-Crofts, 1972.

Hurst, J. Willis. "The Art and Science of Presenting a Patient's Problems." *Archives of Internal Medicine,* 128 (September, 1971), 463-465.

Judge, Richard and Zuidema, George. *Physical Diagnosis: A Physiologic Approach to the Clinical Examination.* Boston: Little, Brown and Company, 1974.

Krause, Marie V. and Hunseher, Martha A. *Food Nutrition and Diet Therapy.* Philadelphia: W.B. Saunders Company, 1972.

Little, Dolores E. and Carnevali, Doris L. *Nursing Care Planning.* Philadelphia: J.B. Lippincott Company, 1969, 69-86.

Litz, Theodore. *The Person: His Development Throughout the Life Cycle.* New York: Basic Books Inc., 1968.

Luckman, Joan and Sorensen, Karen C. *Medical-Surgical Nursing: A Psychophysiologic Approach.* Philadelphia: W.B. Saunders Company, 1974.

Mahoney, Elizabeth A., Verdisco, Laurie A. and Shortridge, Lillie M. *How to Collect and Record a Health History: A Programmed Instruction.* Preliminary copy for field testing. Columbia University School of Nursing, July, 1974.

Marlow, Dorothy R. *Textbook of Pediatric Nursing.* 4th ed. Philadelphia: W.B. Saunders Company, 1973.

Murray, Jeanne. *Nondirective Interviewing: A Programmed Instruction.* Columbia University School of Nursing, July, 1974.

Prior, John A. and Silberstein, Jack S. *Physical Diagnosis: The History and Examination of the Patient.* 4th ed. Saint Louis: The C.V. Mosby Company, 1973.

Schell, Pamella L. and Campbell, Alla T. "POMR-Not Just Another Way to Chart." *Nursing Outlook,* 20 (August, 1972), 510-514.

Stein, Jess F., ed. *The Random House Dictionary of the English Language.* New York: Random House, 1967.

Stevenson, Ian. *The Diagnostic Interview.* 2nd ed. New York: Harper & Row, Publishers, 1971.

Weed, Lawrence L., *Medical Records, Medical Evaluation and Patient Care,* The Press of Case Western Reserve University, 1970. Chap. 1-3 (pp. 16, 18—components of data base).

Wintrobe, Maxwell et al. *Harrison's Textbook of Internal Medicine.* 7th ed. New York: McGraw-Hill Book Company, 1974.

Woody, M. and Mallison, M. "The Problem Oriented System for Patient-Centered Care." *American Journal of Nursing,* 73 (July, 1973), 1168-1175.

"Health Assessment Part I: Health History." Herbert A. Lehman College Department of Nursing.

"Outline Guide for Medical Histories." Columbia University, Presbyterian Hospital.

"Patient Assessment: Taking a Patient's History." Programmed instruction. *American Journal of Nursing,* 74 (February, 1974), 293-324.

iNdEx

Page numbers appearing in *italics*
refer to charts